# Multiple Sclerosis

## The Guide to Treatment
## and Management

# Multiple Sclerosis

## The Guide to Treatment and Management

### 5th Edition

**Chris H. Polman, MD, PhD**
Professor of Neurology
Free University Medical Centre, Amsterdam

**Alan J. Thompson, MD, FRCP, FRCPI**
Garfield Weston Professor of Clinical Neurology and Neurorehabilitation
Institute of Neurology, Queen Square, University College, London

**T. Jock Murray, OC, MD, FRCPC, MACP, FRCP**
Professor of Medicine (Neurology)
Professor of Medical Humanities
Dalhousie University, Halifax, Nova Scotia

**W. Ian McDonald, MB, PhD, FRCP, FMedSci**
Professor of Clinical Neurology (Emeritus)
Institute of Neurology, Queen Square, London

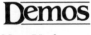

New York

Demos Medical Publishing, Inc., 386 Park Avenue South, New York, New York 10016

Library of Congress Cataloging-in-Publication Data is available from the publisher upon request and on our web site: www.demosmedpub.com

ISBN: 1-888799-54-4



Printed in Canada

# Contents

# Preface

Since publication of the fourth edition of *Therapeutic Claims in Multiple Sclerosis* in 1996, the ability to modify the course of the disease has changed the outlook of people with multiple sclerosis (MS). There now are grounds for hope that still more effective treatments than those we have at present will soon be developed.

An equally important development has been the improvement in symptomatic management and neurologic rehabilitation. New drugs have been developed, and more effective ways of administering older drugs have been devised. Controlled trials of certain aspects of neurorehabilitation have shown that this is an effective approach to management.

This book provides a comprehensive, readily accessible guide to the wide diversity of therapeutic options now available to treat MS. As with previous editions, all therapies in current use are discussed in detail and an opinion statement is given for each that reflects consensus opinion about its usefulness and effectiveness.

In deciding whether to adopt a particular form of treatment (whether it be medical, surgical, rehabilitative, or "alternative"), it is necessary to weigh the evidence about effectiveness and the risk and nature of side effects. We have done that in this book to the best of our ability, and wherever possible we have based our recommendations on scientific, peer-reviewed publications.

Readers of the previous editions of this book will notice that we have provided a guide to further reading to which they can refer to obtain additional details about particular treatments and how their effectiveness and side effects have been assessed. Readers who wish to obtain summaries or abstracts of the journal articles cited in this book may find them by "Medline" searches, available through the website of the National Library of Medicine (www.hlm.nih.gov); the entire articles may be obtained from medical libraries.

The Internet is the first place to which many people now turn for information. Accordingly, in addition to publishing the book in print form, its content is available on the Multiple Sclerosis International Federation's web site, "The World of MS," (www.msinternational. org). The online version will allow for rapid updating of material between print editions, and we urge readers to use this resource to access newly available information

All material included in this volume was reviewed by members of the Medical Management Committee, all of whom are neurologists in active practice who treat patients with MS on a daily basis; the authors thank them for their many suggestions and comments. Their opinions are based not only on published data but also on their daily experiences and information from trusted colleagues. We give special thanks to the Multiple Sclerosis International Federation (London), the official sponsor of this volume, for facilitating publication of the fifth edition.

# Foreword

Thanks to the Internet, information about multiple sclerosis has never been more widely available. It has enabled people affected by MS and health professionals in every part of the world to share their knowledge about effective treatments and has created a real opportunity for truly international cooperation in finding a cure and ending the devastating effects of this disease.

However, this rich source of facts, advice, and support is tempered by the fact that the Internet also holds a vast amount of misinformation and opinion. It has become increasingly important, therefore, to deliver up-to-date and accurate information in order to distinguish valid treatments from those that are ineffective or even dangerous.

The Multiple Sclerosis International Federation (MSIF) prides itself on distributing quality information on all aspects of MS and is particularly pleased to publish this fifth edition of the book previously called *Therapeutic Claims in Multiple Sclerosis*. It is the result of meticulous work by the International Medical Advisory Board of the MSIF to establish authoritative guidance on a wide range of therapies currently being used in the management of MS. The book has been completely revised and restructured with conclusions based on the latest research.

People with MS, their friends and caregivers, and, of course, health professionals will find great value in the *Guide*, and the MSIF thanks everyone who has contributed so generously of his or her time to produce this edition. I commend *Multiple Sclerosis: The Guide to Treatment and Management* to you as *the* book to read on MS therapies.

Christine Purdy
Chief Executive
Multiple Sclerosis
International Federation
January 2001

# MSIF Medical Management Committee

Dr. Fernando Cáceres
*Beruti 3737 6 to 22*
*Buenos Aires, Argentina*

Professor Michel Clanet
*Hôpital Purpan*
*Place du Docteur Baylac*
*Toulouse, France*

Prof. H-P Hartung
*Professor and Chairman*
*Department of Neurology*
*Karl-Franzens-Universitat Graz*
*Graz, Austria*

Professor Jürg Kesselring
*Rheuma und Rehazentrum*
*Department of Neurology*
*Valens, Switzerland*

Dr. Liz McDonald
*Multiple Sclerosis Society*
*Victoria, Australia*

Professor W. Ian McDonald
*Professor (Emeritus), University Department of Clinical Neurology*
*The National Hospital, Queen Square*
*London, England*

# CHAPTER 1

# Introduction

The last years of the twentieth century witnessed a transformation in the way we think about multiple sclerosis (MS). From the neurologist's perspective, although important gaps in our knowledge remain, we understand better the way in which the nervous system is damaged by the disease and how symptoms are produced. These advances led to new approaches to treatment, and the first successful steps have been taken.

For the first time, the ability to modify the course of the disease has changed the outlook of people with MS. There now are grounds for hope—that the course of the disease can be modified, that symptoms can be alleviated, and that more effective treatments than those we have at present treatments will soon be developed.

The huge expansion of information available about MS, not least on the Internet, has put the individual with MS in a position to take increasing responsibility for her or his own care. There is thus a need for a comprehensive, readily accessible guide to the present therapeutic options, which will give the inquirer a balanced guide to the relative effectiveness of individual treatments.

This book is designed to do just that.

The Internet is the first place to which many people now turn for information. Accordingly, as well as publishing the book in print form, we

1

have placed it on the International Federation of MS Society's web site, "The World of MS" <www.msinternational.org>. The online version will allow for rapid updating of material between print editions.

Scientific advances relevant to MS have occurred in a number of fields. Unquestionably the largest single contribution has been from the exploitation of magnetic resonance techniques, both magnetic resonance imaging (MRI) and magnetic resonance spectroscopy (MRS).

The serial use of such methods has shown that disease activity often is 10 times more frequent than had been suspected from simply recording relapse rate. In turn, this observation has led to the development of methods to screen quickly treatments that are designed to reduce the frequency of new damage in the central nervous system.

The use of special MR techniques has led to a new understanding of how the damage evolves. The development of a new lesion most often is heralded by a focal area of "breakdown" of the barrier that normally exists between the blood and the brain; this is associated with immunologically mediated inflammation. Demyelination (the characteristic pathologic change in MS) occurs at approximately the same time. The inflammation subsides after about a month, and the early phase recovery mechanisms are expressed, leading to clinical recovery (i.e., remission.). But, of course, neurologic deficit accumulates in most people with MS, leading to disability as time goes by.

A recent development with potential therapeutic implications is the realization that an important factor contributing to the irrecoverable component of disability is complete degeneration of the nerve fibers.

As so often happens when powerful new techniques are introduced, unexpected complexity is revealed. For example, there is now evidence that not all MS lesions have a detectable inflammatory component; this is particularly true in the form of MS that progresses inexorably from onset without clear-cut relapses and remissions (primary progressive MS). However, this is also true for some lesions in other forms of MS. In addition, there is increasing evidence that what appears on MRI to be normal white matter in the brain often contains abnormalities in structure and chemical composition.

These new insights suggest new strategies for treatment, and more than 80 agents are being assessed at the beginning of the twenty-first century.

It has already been mentioned that MR methods have speeded up the process of determining whether a treatment is effective in reducing disease activity. However, establishing the nature of the relationship between disease activity as judged by MRI and disability has proved to be very difficult. For this reason, it is still necessary to demonstrate effectiveness using clinical measures. This previously was done by means of the large, double-blind, placebo-controlled clinical trial.

Here we confront a problem born of the very success of these approaches in recent years. Such trials have shown that it is possible to modify the course of the disease with two classes of agents that are now licensed for use, at least in some countries—the beta-interferons and glatiramer acetate. Given that partially effective treatment is available, it can no longer be ethically justified to carry out placebo-controlled clinical trials on a large scale and over a long period, which has been necessary so far to demonstrate the effectiveness of these agents.

Shorter term trials might be justified, but they are likely to have limited application in a disease with such a prolonged time course as MS. A new treatment can be compared with an existing treatment, but a trial designed to do this is much more difficult to interpret than a placebo-controlled trial and inevitably is even more expensive. Clearly, a new approach is needed, and this is the current focus of an international collaborative project being organized under the auspices of the International Federation of Multiple Sclerosis Societies.

So far we have dealt with treatments designed to modify the course of the disease. An equally important development during the last decade or so is the improvement in symptomatic management and neurologic rehabilitation. New drugs have been developed, and more effective ways of administering older drugs have been devised. Controlled trials of certain aspects of neurorehabilitation have shown that this is an effective approach to management.

## Evidence of Effectiveness and the Selection of Treatment

Two problems pervade all aspects of treatment of MS, as well as other serious and highly variable chronic diseases. First is the problem of establishing effectiveness, and second is that of demonstrating that the chance of obtaining benefit outweighs the risk of unwanted side effects. The latter point is important because many drugs that influence the nervous system or the immune system have side effects that may be serious. The particular problem in MS is that, with the tendency to virtually complete remission early in the course of the disease and the wide variations in intervals between relapses (we have seen a number of examples of more than 30 years), it is very difficult to know whether improvement in the clinical state or a period of several years without a relapse is a consequence of the treatment used or if it was going to happen anyway. The double-blind, placebo-controlled clinical trial was developed to overcome this problem, which applies equally to orthodox medical, surgical, and rehabilitative treatments and to "alternative" therapies. Another aspect of treatment is the enormous cost involved in prescribing some of the newer drugs. Increasing attention is being devoted to issues of cost-effectiveness, although its measurement is still a controversial matter.

The selection of a treatment for a symptom or for a disease or as a preventative measure should be a decision that is based on evidence that it is safe and effective.

There are different levels of evidence. A neighbor's claim that some medicine helped her or stories of someone who responded dramatically to a therapy (anecdotal evidence) constitute weak evidence. More people claiming the same thing adds weight but still is not solid evidence, since almost any approach—useful or useless—has enthusiastic believers.

The fact that something has been around for many years, or even centuries, also is not very strong evidence. There are many examples, such as bleeding, which were used for thousands of years. We now know that it probably made people weaker and was sometimes very dangerous and deadly when a person was very sick—and that is when they were often bled more. Nevertheless, it was a widely used and trusted treatment from ancient times up to the twentieth century.

Stronger evidence would be provided by a carefully followed group of patients in an *open trial*—one in which both the physician and the patient know they are using the drug.

Designing a trial of how patients will be treated and assessed over a future time—a *prospective trial*—is stronger evidence than looking back at a group of patients treated in the past to see how they fared—a *retrospective trial*. In open trials, the results often seem better than they really are for a number of reasons. There is the positive bias of the therapist, who wants to see that the patients are better. There is the placebo response of patients, who want to get better and feel good about being in a treatment program for their illness. Additionally, those who do not do well or feel worse stop the treatment, so the therapist accumulates good responders, deals mostly with those who do well, and has the impression that most treated patients do well.

Trials can be made stronger by using a placebo control for comparison and having the treated group and the placebo group matched for as many factors as possible (age, sex, duration, type and severity of disease, etc.) and by keeping both the therapist and the patients "blinded" to whether they are receiving treatment or placebo. This is a randomized, *double-blind, placebo-controlled* trial. The statisticians can indicate how large and how long such a trial should continue to answer the questions being asked in the study. Such a trial provides strong evidence.

Perhaps even stronger evidence comes from a *meta-analysis*, which takes all the well-designed controlled trials and analyzes their results to reach a conclusion about the safety and effectiveness of a treatment.

Information on studies of conventional and alternative approaches are collected and evaluated by the Cochrane Controlled Trials Register, which currently lists 4,000 completed randomized controlled trials of alternative medicine with an equal number in the process of being assessed. There are over 200 systematic reviews of alternative interventions, 40 of which have been assessed in detail and are available from the Cochrane Library web site. http://hiru.mcmaster.ca/COCHRANE/default.htm

Dr. Marcia Angell and Dr. Jerome Kassirer, former editors of the *New England Journal of Medicine*, wrote that there cannot be two kinds of medicine—conventional and alternative: "There is only medicine that has been adequately tested and medicine that has not, medicine that works and medicine that may or may not work." They argued that alternative therapies have been given a free ride, and when something is tested rigorously and shown to be safe and effective it does not matter whether it is alternative or conventional, "but assertions, speculation, and testimonials do not substitute for evidence." They conclude, "Alternative treatments should be subjected to scientific testing no less rigorous than that required for conventional treatments."

In deciding whether to adopt a particular form of treatment (whether it be medical, surgical, rehabilitative, or "alternative"), it is necessary to weigh the evidence about effectiveness and the risk and nature of side effects. We have done that in this book to the best of our ability, and wherever possible we have based our recommendations on scientific, peer-reviewed publications.

We do not consider it to be within our province to comment on cost-effectiveness, which is difficult to measure and is influenced by local variability in the way health care is provided. The exception to this is in

Chapter 5, which considers alternative therapies, both because these are not strictly related to the environment in which medical care is provided and because many of these nonmedical therapies are expensive relative to any real benefit.

A major change from previous editions of this book is the inclusion of a guide to further reading to which the reader can refer to obtain additional details about particular treatments and how their effectiveness and side effects have been assessed.

# CHAPTER 2

# Treatment for an Acute Exacerbation

## Overview

At least 80 to 85 percent of people with MS have an acute period of worsening (also called an exacerbation, bout, attack, or relapse) at some time. One of the most commonly used definitions of an exacerbation is the [sub]acute appearance of a neurologic abnormality that must be present for at least 24 hours in the absence of fever or infection. A wide variety of symptoms can occur during exacerbations. Magnetic resonance imaging (MRI) scans taken at such times often show new active (gadolinium-enhancing) lesions in the brain or the reactivation or enlargement of old lesions. Although almost all relapses remit spontaneously, most clinicians advise treatment for those relapses that have significant functional impact.

Corticosteroids have been the mainstay of treatment for the management of acute relapses for many years. They have immunomodulatory and antiinflammatory effects that restore the integrity of the blood–brain barrier, reduce edema, and possibly facilitate remyelination and improve axonal conduction. Corticosteroid therapy has been shown to shorten the duration and severity of the relapse and accelerate recovery, but there is no convincing evidence that the overall degree of recovery is improved or that the long-term course of the disease is altered.

Adrenocorticotropic hormone (ACTH, corticotropin) was the first agent demonstrated to be helpful in recovery from acute exacerbations. Brief courses of high-dose intravenous (IV) methylprednisolone (IVMP, 500–1000 mg/day for 3–5 days) have generally supplanted ACTH because of convenience, reliability, fewer side effects, and perhaps a more consistent and rapid onset of action.

Results of the Optic Neuritis Treatment Trial have been extrapolated by many neurologists to MS-associated relapses in general. In this study, 457 patients with acute optic neuritis were randomly assigned to receive 1000 mg of IVMP per day for 3 days followed by 1 mg of oral prednisone per kilogram per day for 11 days, 1 mg of oral prednisone per kilogram per day for 14 days, or oral placebo. The advantage of studying cases of optic neuritis is that very sensitive outcome measures (e.g., visual field, contrast sensitivity, color vision, and visual acuity) can be applied. The rate of recovery of vision was significantly faster in the IVMP-treated group, with the greatest benefits in patients with visual acuity of 20/40 or worse at entry. After six months there was no significant difference in visual acuity between the IVMP and placebo groups. Oral prednisone provided no benefit over placebo.

Unanticipated findings were that during the 6 to 24 months of follow-up, the risk of recurrent optic neuritis in either eye was increased with oral prednisone and that IVMP reduced by approximately 50 percent the risk of a new attack leading to the diagnosis of MS. This effect was most evident for patients at highest risk for subsequent relapse, that is, those with multiple brain lesions on MRI at entry into the study. These results should be interpreted with the understanding that this study was not designed to assess the effect of glucocorticoids on subsequent relapses and that the IVMP group was unblinded and lacked a placebo control. Differences between the treatment groups were no longer significant after three years, which suggests that IVMP at best delayed but did not stop the development of MS.

Magnetic resonance imaging follow-up studies have convincingly shown the effect of steroids, as evidenced by the reduction of gadolinium-enhancing lesions; however, this effect is only short-lived, and new enhancing lesions can develop within a week following treatment.

Despite the widespread use of corticosteroids as a treatment for relapses, very little is known about the optimal treatment regimen. The main controversies relate to the relative efficacy of the type of steroid (i.e., intramuscular ACTH vs. IV steroids vs. oral steroids), the optimal dosage for each route of administration, and whether a short course of IV treatment should be followed by a tapering regimen of orally administered corticosteroids.

Some clinicians substitute oral corticosteroid treatment for IVMP for the management of relapses mainly because of its easier route and reduced expense of administration. Data substantiating its equivalent benefit in acute relapse have been presented but are not very persuasive. Remarkably, in various studies—all being rather small—quite different dosage regimens of oral steroids have been applied.

Other antiinflammatory drugs, the so-called nonsteroidal antiinflammatory drugs (NSAIDs), including aspirin, indomethacin, ibuprofen, and naproxen, have not been shown to be of benefit in the treatment of MS relapses.

**Conclusion:** *A short course of IVMP remains the intervention of choice in patients with an acute exacerbation that warrants treatment. Prospective evidence indicates that it diminishes acute neurologic dysfunction; an effect on the long-term course of the disease has not been firmly established. It is unclear whether on oral taper of steroids would add any benefit.*

## Specific Agents

### Intravenous Methylprednisolone

As noted previously, it is common practice to employ a short course of corticosteroids to treat acute relapses of MS. Of the various approaches applied, the administration of IV methylprednisolone (IVMP) has become the most popular, especially because it can be given as a short course (typically 3–5 days), has a rapid onset of action, and is associated with relatively few side effects. Its use is now common practice in many clinics and hospitals, even on an outpatient basis. It should be given only under close medical supervision because side effects, even though extremely rare, include psychosis, peptic ulceration, aseptic bone necrosis, infections, cardiac arrhythmias, and thromboembolism.

Some neurologists also employ periodic pulses of IVMP (e.g., once monthly) in patients with progressive MS, but there is no firm evidence that this has a favorable impact on the course of the disease, and there is an increased risk of side effects.

*In the opinion of the Committee, this treatment can be recommended for patients with exacerbations who have significant functional impact. Long-term use may be associated with significant serious side effects.*

## Intravenous Dexamethasone

Dexamethasone is another corticosteroid that shares many characteristics with methylprednisolone. Although the number of patients with MS exacerbations being treated with IV dexamethasone is substantially smaller than that being treated with IVMP, there is some evidence that its effects are comparable when given as a short course. In many countries its cost is substantially lower than that of IVMP.

*In the opinion of the Committee, it is difficult to give a recommendation in the absence of carefully performed studies, but intravenous dexamethasone may represent a less expensive alternative to treatment with intravenous methylprednisolone; it is no longer available in some countries (e.g., the United Kingdom).*

## Intramuscular Adrenocorticotropic Hormone

Thirty years ago, short-term intramuscular (IM) adrenocorticotropic hormone ACTH given daily in high doses was shown to reduce the severity and shorten the duration of exacerbations. In more recent studies, claims have been made that IVMP works more quickly and effectively than ACTH, and most neurologists now prefer this treatment.

*In the opinion of the Committee, intramuscular ACTH, although proven efficacious, is no longer the preferred treatment for MS exacerbations.*

## Oral Steroids

There is conflicting evidence regarding the efficacy of oral steroids in the treatment of exacerbations. In the optic neuritis study referred to previously, there were more relapses in subsequent months in the oral prednisone group than in either the placebo-treated or the IVMP-treated group. Many people who have examined these data, however, reject the conclusion of the authors that oral prednisone was responsible for the increased later exacerbation rate.

A recent Danish study demonstrated the efficacy of oral methylprednisolone (MP) as a treatment for exacerbations. It compared the effects of oral MP therapy and placebo in patients with an episode lasting less than 4 weeks. Twenty-five patients received placebo, and 26 patients were given 500 mg oral MP once a day for 5 days, followed by a 10-day drug tapering period. Patients receiving MP did consistently better than those receiving placebo. At 8 weeks after the start of treatment, 32 percent of patients in the placebo group had improved by one Expanded Disability Status Scale (EDSS) point, whereas 65 percent of patients taking MP had a similar improvement.

A recent controlled study in the United Kingdom compared oral MP with IVMP: 80 patients with MS were treated within four weeks of the start of an exacerbation. Of these patients, 38 received IVMP (1000 mg/day for 3 days) and 42 received oral MP (48 mg/day for 7 days, followed by 24 mg/day for 7 days and 12 mg/day for the final 7 days). Hence, the cumulative dose of methylprednisolone was 3000 mg in the IV group and 588 mg in the oral group. The primary outcome was the difference between the two groups in improvement in the EDSS score of at least one full point after four weeks. No significant difference was found either with respect to this primary outcome or in any other measurement at any stage of the study. The main concerns regarding this study is that there only was a modest effect of treatment in both arms and that therefore a statistical type II error (real difference not being detected) is quite likely to occur. One must remember in this respect that statistical methods are tools that are predominantly developed to detect differences rather than to prove similarities: the absence of proof of difference is not equal to the proof of absence of difference.

It is extremely important that oral treatment with steroids not be prolonged because the complications of long-term treatment are well established. Complications include generalized puffiness, "moon face," psychosis, peptic ulceration, infections, and acne. Long-term use may even result in serious side effects such as fractures related to bone softening, aseptic necrosis of bone, cataracts, hypertension, and adrenal insufficiency.

*In the opinion of the Committee, treatment with oral steroids, even though it has recently gained some support, is not the preferred treatment for exacerbations because only rather small studies (applying very different dosages) have been performed and it is not clear whether oral treatment, which in many regimens has to be prescribed longer than intravenous treatment, might increase the risk of side effects.*

## Intrathecal Steroids

*In the opinion of the Committee, this therapy should not be used because of reported harmful effects.*

## Aspirin (Sodium Salicylate) and Nonsteroidal Antiinflammatory Drugs (Indomethacin, Phenylbutazone, Naproxen, Ibuprofen, Fenoprofen)

These drugs are widely used to reduce inflammation, especially in arthritis. Proper evaluation of this type of drug in MS has not been done. Small studies, however, suggest that indomethacin might worsen MS and that ibuprofen is safe, although not effective, in reducing the volume of active MS lesions on MRI. Ibuprofen and aspirin are being used to reduce early flulike side effects of interferon beta and appear to be safe for the relief of discomfort.

*In the opinion of the Committee, there appears to be no scientific basis for use of this therapy other than for the relief of early side effects associated with interferon therapy.*

## Plasmapheresis

During plasmapheresis (plasma exchange, or PE), blood is removed from the patient, and the liquid plasma and the cells are separated by centrifuge. The plasma (including many lymphocytes) is discarded and replaced by normal plasma or human albumin to avoid loss of protein and fluid. The "reconstituted" blood is then returned to the patient. This process may be repeated a number of times. It is believed that substances that can damage myelin and/or impair nerve conduction are removed in this way.

There remain numerous reports (most of them uncontrolled and reporting on only very small numbers of patients) that PE may be effective in fulminant acute syndromes of MS (or acute disseminated encephalomyelitis).

*In the opinion of the Committee, this therapy might be considered only for those rare cases that present with acute, fulminant symptomatology and do not respond to intravenous steroids.*

# Guide to Further Reading

- Milligan NG, Newcombe R, Compston DAS. A double-blind controlled trial of high dose methylprednisolone in patients with multiple sclerosis. 1. Clinical effects. *J Neurol Neurosurg Psychiatry* 1986; 50:511–516.
- Thompson AJ, Kennard C, Swash M, et al. Relative efficacy of intravenous methylprednisolone and ACTH in the treatment of acute relapse in MS. *Neurology* 1989; 39:969–971.
- Beck RW, Cleary PA, Anderson MM, et al. A randomized, controlled trial of corticosteroids in the treatment of acute optic neuritis. The Optic Neuritis Study Group. *N Engl J Med* 1992; 326:581–588.
- Beck RW, Cleary PA, Trobe JD, et al. The effect of corticosteroids for acute optic neuritis on the subsequent development of multiple sclerosis. The Optic Neuritis Study Group. *N Engl J Med* 1993; 329:1764–1769.
- Barnes D, Hughes RAC, Morris RW, et al. Randomised trial of oral and intravenous methylprednisolone in acute relapses of multiple sclerosis. *Lancet* 1997; 349:902–906.
- Sellebjerg F, Frederiksen JL, Nielsen PM, Olesen J. Double-blind, randomized, placebo-controlled study of oral, high-dose methylprednisolone in attacks of MS. *Neurology* 1998; 51:529–534.
- Weinshenker BG, O'Brien PC, Petterson TM, et al. A randomized trial of plasma exchange in acute central nervous system inflammatory demyelinating disease. *Ann Neurol* 1999; 46:878–886.

# CHAPTER 3

# Treatments That Affect the Long-Term Course of the Disease ("Disease-Modifying Therapy")

The goal of therapy in patients with MS is to prevent relapses and progressive worsening of the disease. The documentation of therapeutic advances in MS is dependent on large, randomized, controlled clinical trials because of the highly variable and unpredictable course of the disease and the difficulty in precisely measuring neurologic disability.

Immunosuppressive drugs that dampen most or certain aspects of immune system function were used initally, but they have never found widespread acceptance because of the fact that various studies have met with limited success as a result of variable efficacy and considerable toxicity (especially with long-term use), mainly because of the induction of bone marrow suppression.

More recently, large, randomized, controlled trials have been performed with substances that should be seen as immune *modulators* rather than immune *suppressors*. Such studies at this moment have led to the regulatory approval of four agents [Avonex®, Betaseron® (Betaferon® in Europe), Copaxone®, and Rebif®] for reducing the severity and frequency of relapses. More recently, data have been published that suggest that Betaferon® might also have a favorable impact on the disease once it has entered the secondary progressive phase, the phase that is characterized by gradual accrual of disability. Although there is some evidence for a reduction in the rate of progression of neurologic impairment and disability, none of these agents have been shown to achieve a sustained remission, complete halt of further progression, or substantial alleviation of long-standing disability.

Therefore, in individual patients, decisions to initiate treatment should be based on the course of that patient's disease. On the one hand, approximately 10 to 20 percent of patients have relatively benign disease, so not every patient may require disease-modifying therapy. On the other hand, one should not postpone treatment until after persistent neurologic deficits have occurred because none of the available compounds reverse fixed deficits. Disease-modifying therapy should be considered early in the course for patients with an unfavorable prognosis, but, unfortunately, the rate and pattern of progression of disease cannot be reliably predicted at initial assessment. Although long-term follow-up of monosymptomatic patients indicates that the likelihood of a second clinical event and that of the development of disability increases with certain clinical characteristics (progressive course of disease, sphincter or motor symptoms at onset, male sex, high attack frequency within the first years) as well as with the lesion load on brain MRI, determining the exact future prospectives for a given individual is still not possible because the prognostic value of these factors is only modest.

Before long-term therapies are implemented, it is extremely important that counseling about realistic objectives, regarding both efficacy and side effects, take place because overly optimistic expectations may complicate treatment.

## From Better Understanding to Better Treatment

Although the cause of MS is not known, it is generally believed that environmental factors (possibly viral infections) trigger an immunologically mediated process in individuals of a certain genetic background. Genetic factors involved in disease susceptibility probably consist of multiple interacting genes.

Because current theories favor the idea that MS is an immunologic disease, a brief review of the immune system is important. The normal function of the immune system is to recognize and repel foreign invaders, such as bacteria, viruses, and other foreign substances (antigens). It normally is careful to recognize "self" components and not destroy them by mistake. An "autoimmune" disease occurs when this system fails to recognize a "self" component as such and attacks it; in the case of MS, strong evidence points to a mistaken attack on myelin, which surrounds most neurons.

Almost 60 years ago it was shown that injections of brain extracts in animals would make some of them develop an inflammatory disease of the central nervous system (CNS) called experimental allergic encephalomyelitis (EAE). EAE was quite similar to a disease accidentally produced in some humans with an old preparation of rabies vaccine that contained fragments of myelin. Post–rabies vaccine encephalomyelitis, in turn, was quite similar pathologically to occasional forms of postinfectious encephalomyelitis appearing in a few unlucky children after naturally occurring measles, rubella, chickenpox, and occasionally other viruses.

Postinfectious encephalomyelitis in humans is not a recurrent disease; it occurs only once. Later it was shown that a chronic relapsing form of EAE could be produced in some genetically susceptible animals; these animals recovered from attacks of paralysis only to develop symptoms weeks or months later in a manner similar to development of MS symptoms. Moreover, pathologic changes in the CNS in such animals are much like those seen in MS.

However, there are important differences between MS and chronic EAE. Antibodies to myelin proteins are difficult to find in the blood of MS patients, in contrast to EAE. In EAE the antigen is clearly myelin or a myelin component; in MS the antigen is still unknown. Another important difference is that EAE is easily inhibited and suppressed by a number of drugs that seem to have little impact on MS.

The immune system is complex. Its basic units are two kinds of white blood cells located in the thymus, spleen, and lymph nodes. These cells circulate to all parts of the body by way of the blood and the lymph. The larger cells are *macrophages* (Greek: "big-eaters"). They function by engulfing and disposing of debris; they also secrete chemicals known as proteases, which are capable of destroying myelin, prostaglandins, and free oxygen radicals, which have profound effects on inflammation and immune function. The smaller cells are *lymphocytes*, which come in several varieties. *B lymphocytes* are processed in the bone marrow and become antibody-producing cells. The more numerous *T lymphocytes* are processed mostly in the thymus gland; they become activated when exposed to an antigen to which they are reactive; the cell becomes metabolically more active, enlarges, and secretes a group of chemicals called *cytokines*; some of the functions of cytokines are to promote enlargement of lymphocyte populations, activate macrophages, increase blood flow and edema of tissue, and attract other types of white blood cells to the area. Interferon gamma is one such cytokine secreted by activated T cells; it is a substance that facilitates antigen recognition; its use in the treatment of MS has been associated with an increase in the frequency of exacerbations.

Current evidence suggests that cytokines can basically be divided into *proinflammatory* cytokines, such as tumor necrosis factor (TNF-alpha), and interferon gamma (IFN-gamma), which may be directly responsible for tissue damage in MS, and *antiinflammatory* cytokines, such as interleukin-4 (IL-4), interleukin-10 (IL-10), and transforming growth factor beta (TGF-beta), which suppress or inhibit disease.

Many B lymphocytes also exist in and around the MS plaques, but they are relatively uncommon in the cerebrospinal fluid (CSF); they are the source of local immunoglobulin production. Immunoglobulins are antibodies, but in the case of MS the target antigen is unknown, and efforts to find the antigen by studying the antibodies have been largely unsuccessful so far.

It has been clearly established from neuropathologic studies of MS lesions that it is against this background of inflammatory cells and cytokines that active demyelination takes place. Traditionally, inflammation and demyelination are considered to be the hallmark of MS lesions (MS is often listed as an "inflammatory demyelinating disease"); recent studies, however, have reemphasized the importance of damage of neural cells themselves ("axonal damage") as a major correlate of permanent clinical deficits.

Therapeutic approaches aim at utilizing the increased level of understanding of the immune system, for example, by administering antiinflammatory cytokines to patients with MS or by developing strategies that inhibit proinflammatory cytokines. However, the complex network of the immune system with mutually interdependent factors and mechanisms, which can vary between different phases of the disease, limits the ability to predict the effect of an immune intervention once given to a patient. Additional complexity is introduced by the emerging pathologic heterogeneity of MS that apparently encompasses a spectrum from highly destructive cellular lesions, demyelinative processes with or without significant cellular involvement, to primary oligodendrogliopathies.

Given our limited understanding of disease pathogenesis in general and in a given person with the disease, concrete therapeutic advances in

MS are critically dependent on clinical trials. Because of the highly variable and unpredictable course of the disease and the difficulty in precisely measuring neurologic disability, these trials traditionally require large numbers of patients and long periods of follow-up.

## Drugs Approved for Use in MS

### Interferon Beta (Avonex®, Betaseron®/Betaferon®, and Rebif®)

Interferons (IFNs) are small molecules (cytokines) produced by cells of the immune system in response to a variety of inducers, especially viruses. They have been demonstrated to have antiviral, antiproliferative, and immunomodulating properties and are divided into two types: type 1 includes alpha and beta IFN, whereas type 2 is gamma IFN. IFNs were initially considered for the treatment of MS because of a presumed viral pathogenesis. Because there was some evidence for a decrease in the level of IFN gamma in the CSF of MS patients, a pilot study was performed to assess its safety and efficacy. This trial was prematurely terminated because of an unexpected increase in the relapse rate. The negative result of this trial provided an important clue to the understanding of the pathogenesis of MS, and subsequent studies focused on the effects of type 1 IFNs because they were found to have a number of immunomodulatory effects that were quite the opposite of those of IFN gamma. IFN alpha and beta use the same receptor and have similar effects and a high degree of homology.

A number of smaller studies have reported limited efficacy for intrathecally, subcutaneously, and intramuscularly administered type 1 IFN in decreasing the frequency of exacerbations in relapsing-remitting MS. In some of these studies, these effects were shown to be reversible, with the return of markers of disease activity to baseline after discontinuation of treatment. This supported the hypothesis that the observed changes were indeed the result of IFN therapy. Therefore, further studies were performed, which took advantage of the availability of recombinant IFN and abandoned natural IFN. At present, two forms of recombinant IFN beta (1a and 1b) have been approved by regulatory authorities. Both are made by recombinant DNA technology in tissue culture and are highly purified before use. IFN beta-1a is a glycosylated, recombinant mammalian-cell product, with an amino acid sequence identical to that of natural interferon beta. IFN beta-1b is a nonglycosylated recombinant bacterial-cell product in which serine is substituted for cysteine at position 17.

## Interferon Beta-1a

Two forms of IFN beta-1a were subject to investigation in large clinical trials: Avonex® and Rebif®. Avonex® was tested in a trial involving 301 patients with relapsing MS and mild to moderate neurologic impairment (baseline disability score on the EDSS 1.0–3.5). Treatment consisted of weekly intramuscular (IM) injections (6 million units, or 30 mcg) or placebo for up to two years, the dose and timing of administration being based on the serum level of beta$_2$-microglobulin and the occurrence of side effects. The principal outcome measure was the length of time to progression of disability, defined as a worsening from baseline of at least one point on the EDSS that persisted for at least 6 months.

The study was prematurely terminated when it was recognized that the drop-out rate was less than anticipated. At the time the trial was stopped, 57 percent of enrolled patients had completed two years, and 77 percent had been followed up for 18 months. Despite this early termination, IFN beta-1a–treated patients were significantly less likely to reach the primary outcome, the probability being about 21 percent in the treatment group and 33 percent in the placebo group for those who completed two years of therapy. An 18 percent reduction in exacerbations was noted for the treated group, and those patients who completed two years had one-third fewer exacerbations. The treatment effect was supported by a reduction of gadolinium enhancement and new or enlarging lesions on annual MRIs; a significant difference between the treatment groups, however, was not found for the total brain lesion load.

The clinical significance of the beneficial effect of IFN beta-1a on disease progression at the lower EDSS scores has been endorsed by the findings of a post hoc statistical analysis of the disability outcomes data obtained in this study. Sensitivity calculations indicated that the primary outcome parameter was robust to changes in definitions of EDSS progression and that the proportion of patients progressing to EDSS milestones of 4.0 and 6.0 was significantly lower in the IFN-treated patients.

Very recent reports indicate that in a placebo-controlled study involving almost 400 individuals with a first episode suggestive for MS and specific MRI features that are prognostically unfavorable, Avonex® significantly prolonged the time to a second episode; full peer-reviewed publication of these data is eagerly awaited.

A large study investigating the effects of Avonex® on disease progression in patients with secondary progressive MS is currently ongoing.

Rebif® was investigated in a number of studies, including one in which 560 patients with active relapsing-remitting disease and mild to moderate disability (EDSS 0–5) were randomized to treatment with IFN beta-1a 6 MIU (22 mcg), 12 MIU (44 mcg), or placebo, given subcutaneously three times a week for two years. The primary end point for this study was the relapse rate. At the end of the study 95 percent of patient data were available for analysis. The results showed that, compared with placebo, IFN beta-1a significantly decreased the number (by 27% and 33% with 22 mcg and 44 mcg, respectively) and severity of exacerbations, increased time to first and second relapses, and increased the percentage of patients who were relapse-free during the study.

In addition, IFN beta-1a prolonged the time to confirmed progression as measured with EDSS scores (1.0 point confirmed at 3 months). Furthermore, there was a significant reduction in the disease activity on MRI (gadolinium-enhancing lesions, new lesions, or enlarging T2 lesions) as well as on total T2 lesion load in patients receiving active treatment compared with those given placebo. The placebo group showed an accumulation of approximately 11 percent in lesion load over the two years, whereas there was a decrease of about 1 percent among patients receiving 6 MIU and a decrease of almost 4 percent in the 12 MIU group. Extended observation of these patients for up to four years has suggested that 44 mcg three times a week is superior to 22 mcg three times a week for some of the outcome measures applied.

Another study with Rebif® compared three different doses of IFN beta-1a administered once weekly with placebo, showing increasing treatment effect with increasing dose, thereby suggesting that some of the currently applied dosage regimens could be improved.

It was reported recently that, in a large placebo-controlled trial in secondary progressive MS, Rebif® given three times weekly failed to have a significant effect on disease progression, as defined by the time to confirmed neurologic deterioration (1-point increase) on the EDSS present for at least three months, and that Rebif® 22 mcg once weekly reduced the likelihood of a second episode in the next two years in patients with a first episode suggestive of MS who have prognostically unfavorable MRI features. So far, the results of these trials have been presented only in abstract form; full publication of the data is eagerly awaited.

## Interferon Beta-1b

Interferon beta-1b was initially tested in a multicenter U.S. trial involving 372 patients with relapsing-remitting MS and mild to moderate disability (EDSS up to 5.5). Treatment consisted of either 8 MIU (250 mcg) or 1.6 MIU (50 mcg) of IFN beta-1b or placebo given by subcutaneous injection every other day. The primary outcome was the relapse rate. Compared with placebo, treatment with the higher dose reduced the relapse rate by 31 percent, increased the time to first relapse and the proportion of patients who were relapse-free, and reduced by about 50 percent the number of patients who had moderate and severe relapses. There was, however, no difference in changes in EDSS scores between treatment groups. The patients in the placebo group had a mean increase of 17 percent in the total lesion load on brain MRI at three years compared with a mean decrease of 6 percent in those receiving high-dose IFN beta-1b. In addition, there was a significant reduction in disease activity as measured by the analysis of new or enlarging lesions on serial MRIs.

A second multicenter trial of IFN beta-1b was performed in Europe and included 718 patients with secondary progressive MS (EDSS at inclusion 3.0–6.5) whose disease had been clinically active in the two years preceding the study (defined as either two relapses or deterioration of at least 1 EDSS point). Treatment consisted of either 8 MIU of IFN beta-1b or placebo subcutaneously on alternate days over three years. The primary outcome was the time to confirmed neurologic deterioration, defined as a 1-point increase on the EDSS present for at least three months. In this study, for EDSS scores of 6.0 and higher a change of 0.5 point was considered to be equal to 1.0 point for scores lower than 6.0. A prospectively planned interim analysis for efficacy was performed after all patients completed at least 24 months of treatment. An alpha level of 0.0133 was predetermined for the intent-to-treat analysis of the primary end point.

Based on this interim analysis, the independent Advisory Board recommended that the study be stopped because there was a highly significant difference regarding the primary end point ($p = 0.0008$). The delay of progression was within a range of 9 to 12 months. This effect was seen in patients both with and without superimposed relapses before or during the study, and it was consistent across all baseline EDSS levels studied. Significant reductions in time to require wheelchair use (EDSS 7.0), number of steroid courses given, and number of MS-related hospitalizations were also observed. Effects on relapse rate and MRI were consistent with the findings in the relapsing-remitting population. Whereas the mean lesion volume increased by about 8 percent at two years, the mean lesion load in the active treatment group decreased by about 5 percent. In a subcohort of patients (n = 125), a marked and significant reduction of new and enhancing lesions could be demonstrated for two six-month periods of frequent scanning (months 1–6 and 19–24).

A recent report suggests that this favorable effect on disability progression could not be confirmed in a North American study of IFN beta-1b in secondary progressive MS. In the absence of a full publication on this study, it is presently impossible to fully understand the discrepancy between both studies.

## SIDE EFFECTS ASSOCIATED WITH INTERFERON BETA TREATMENT

Treatment with IFN beta usually is well tolerated. Side effects depend partially on the dosage used and the route of administration. For all preparations mentioned, patients can experience flulike reactions such as fever, myalgia, chills, and general discomfort for 24 to 48 hours after each injection, especially during the first months of treatment. These symptoms, however, decrease over time, and only few people continue to experience them. Symptom management requires simple practical techniques such as dose escalation, bed-time dosing, and the use of acetaminophen (paracetamol in Europe) or ibuprofen. The frequency of injection-site reactions (redness, tenderness, swelling) is also initially high, almost exclusively in those patients in whom treatment is given by subcutaneous injection, and can be managed by improving injection technique and maintaining site rotation. Injection-site necrosis occurs in about 5 percent of patients. In earlier studies, there was a suggestion that treatment with IFN beta could lead to depression or suicide attempts, but this was not supported by subsequent studies. Some people with MS report an initial worsening of symptoms during the first weeks of IFN therapy; an increase in spasticity has been reported in patients with secondary progressive disease. IFN beta can also cause elevations in liver function tests, lymphopenia, or anemia. Some reports addressed the potential for severe autoimmune disease (thyroiditis, hepatitis) after administration of IFN beta, but a causal relationship has not been convincingly demonstrated so far.

Overall, the percentage of patients discontinuing treatment because of serious or intolerable side effects is low.

UNRESOLVED ISSUES RELATED TO TREATMENT
WITH INTERFERON BETA

Although a number of studies have now provided supportive evidence that IFN beta favorably influences the short-term course of MS, the long-term effects on the development of disability are not known.

Another important consideration is the propensity for IFN beta to stimulate the formation of neutralizing antibodies (NABs), which might depend on a number of variables, including dose administered, route of administration, frequency of administration, and type of IFN beta used. A number of studies suggest that the rate of NAB formation seems to be less in the IFN beta-1a trials (5–20 percent as compared with 25–35 percent for IFN beta-1b), but one must take into account the fact that different assays were used in some of these studies. Initially there were reports that the development of NABs was associated with reduced effectiveness, but concerns regarding the long-term effects of NABs have been somewhat lessened by reanalysis of the initial correlations and recent evidence that they may disappear with long-term treatment. Because of the uncertain validity of the assay of NABs and the limited study of their consequences, clinical decisions based on the presence or absence of NABs cannot yet be made with confidence.

The cost of therapy, currently at least the equivalent of U.S. $10,000, requires a careful cost-benefit analysis. It is still not known when treatment ideally should be initiated or whether it should be discontinued at some point. For individual patients, these costs and the still rather limited information on long-term risks may outweigh the benefits, especially if they have benign disease. The issue of whether long-term therapy should start at the time of the first attack should be reviewed when full reports on both placebo-controlled studies that have recently been completed in this patient population are available; present guidelines for stopping therapy are related to side effects, a desire to become pregnant, and perceived inefficacy as documented by frequent relapses or progression of disability.

Clarifying the mechanism of action also is of great importance, not only because it could guide further research with respect to other treatment modalities that could be used (alone or in combination with IFN beta) but also because it might allow discrimination between those patients who are likely to respond to the drug and those who are not. Mechanisms under consideration include inhibition of T-lymphocyte activation, reduction of IFN gamma and MHC-II expression, increase in IL-

10 production, reduction in blood–brain barrier permeability, and alteration of the body's response to viral infections.

> *In the opinion of the Committee, treatment with interferon beta is the treatment of choice for patients with active relapsing disease. Although the efficacy data are quite robust, the final decision to initiate treatment can be made only in an interaction with an individual patient who is well informed about the consequences of the treatment. At this time it is not possible to decide which, if any, of the interferon beta preparations should be preferred; for patients who respond with severe skin reactions to subcutaneous administration, intramuscular treatment with IFN beta-1a (Avonex®) is recommended. For patients with active (secondary) progressive disease, the recommendation to initiate treatment so far is weak because at the time of this writing it is based on only one published clinical trial (European IFN beta-1b study). The recommendation for secondary progressive disease should be revisited as the detailed results of further trials become available.*

## Glatiramer Acetate (Copaxone®)

Glatiramer acetate (previously called copolymer-1) is a synthetic copolymer, composed of alanine, glutamine, lysine, and tyrosine, with some immunologic similarities to one of the important myelin components, myelin basic protein (MBP), without itself being encephalitogenic. The observation that it inhibits the animal model EAE prompted double-blind clinical trials.

The largest of those was a two-year double-blind trial carried out in the United States and involving 251 patients with relapsing-remitting MS (baseline EDSS 0–5). Treatment consisted of daily subcutaneous injections of 20 mg of glatiramer acetate or placebo. The primary end point was the annualized relapse rate, which was reduced by 29 percent in the group receiving active treatment. There also was a reduction in the percentage of patients remaining relapse-free and the median time to first relapse. A statistically significant favorable effect on EDSS progression was evident only with a less conservative data analysis, thereby providing a trend, but not significant proof for an effect on progression of disability. Awaiting the completion of the analysis of the study, it was extended for a mean of about five months; observations during this extension phase indicate that the clinical benefit of glatiramer acetate was sustained. For some years there has been a lack of MRI data, but recently preliminary data from a nine-month, double-blind, placebo-controlled trial with a primary MRI end point favoring glatiramer acetate have been presented.

Adverse effects of glatiramer acetate are usually mild, including localized injection-site reactions and a systemic reaction occurring within minutes of administration of the drug (associated with chest pain, palpitations, or dyspnea, and always resolving spontaneously in less than 30 minutes). This reaction occurs in a small minority of patients, usually only once, and not necessarily after the first injection.

Serum antibodies to glatiramer acetate also develop, but their presence seems to have no effect on the clinical benefit.

The apparent effect on reducing relapse rate might be due to blocking of the presentation of certain myelin antigens to T lymphocytes.

*In the opinion of the Committee, glatiramer acetate represents an alternative to interferon beta therapy for patients with relapsing-remitting MS. At this time, however, it may be most useful for patients who either are resistant to IFN beta or do not tolerate it because of side effects. Recent suggestions that the drug slows the rate of disability progression need confirmation in additional studies. Glatiramer acetate still has not been licensed in many parts of the world.*

## Treatments That Are Not Specifically Approved for MS But Are Being Used in Certain Parts of the World

A number of other treatment modalities, most of which are accepted treatments for inflammatory, immune-mediated diseases outside the CNS, have also been investigated in MS. Although they have not been licensed for use in MS so far, evidence in favor or against their use is reviewed in this section.

### Intravenous Immunoglobulin

Intravenous immunoglobulin (IVIG) is pooled human IgG that is presumed to alter the immune system by various mechanisms.

Whereas some smaller studies initially failed to reveal clear evidence of efficacy, a more recent Austrian multicenter study provided evidence that monthly administered, low-dose IVIG is effective and well tolerated. A group of 148 patients with relapsing-remitting disease (EDSS 1–6) were randomized to receive monthly doses of IVIG (0.15–0.20 g/kg) or placebo for two years. Primary outcome measures were the effect of treatment on clinical disability, measured by the change in EDSS, and the proportion of patients with improved, stable, or worse disability (at least 1 point on the EDSS scale). Intent-to-treat analysis showed that IVIG had a significant, albeit small, beneficial effect on the EDSS end points; in addition, it reduced relapse rates by about half without having an apparent effect on relapse severity. However, it is possible that blinding was not optimal, and this may have biased the study results. Unfortunately, MRI examinations were not obtained in this study, and no data on three-month or six-month "confirmed" EDSS change were presented.

In another study, an effect of higher doses of IVIG (2.0 g/kg monthly for 6 months) on MRI activity could be established, but in this study there was a high number of drop-outs because of adverse events.

In an Israeli double-blind study of 40 patients with relapsing-remitting MS, people were randomly assigned to receive a loading dose of IVIG (0.4 mg/kg/day for 5 days), followed by single boosters (0.4 mg/kg) or placebo once every two months for two years. Annual exacerbation rate was reduced by about 40 percent, and there was an effect on EDSS scores. However, total lesion score on brain MRI did not show a significant difference between groups.

Severe side effects of treatment with IVIG are uncommon but include aseptic meningitis, renal failure, vascular events, viral infection, eczema, and anaphylaxis. Another potential problem associated with the use of IVIG is that a number of studies have shown that the constituents present in commercially available IVIG preparations can be quite variable.

In addition to having immunoregulatory capacity (by suppressing production of proinflammatory cytokines or by containing anti-idiotypic antibodies), some studies suggest that IVIG might be able to promote remyelination. However, small clinical studies performed at the Mayo Clinic do not support the hypothesis that IVIG might be effective in reversing long-standing neurologic and visual deficits.

*In the opinion of the Committee, the results of the studies that have been published are encouraging. Results of various ongoing studies that determine whether and in what dosage IVIG reduces relapse rate, slows disease progression, or promotes recovery should be awaited before a clear recommendation can be made, and therefore its use is not currently advised.*

## Azathioprine

Azathioprine is an immunosuppressive drug that is widely used in a variety of immune-mediated disorders. A meta-analysis of five double-blind and two single-blind, randomized, controlled trials involving a total of 793 MS patients supported the conclusion that oral azathioprine (1–3 mg/kg/m²) reduces the rate of relapse and might have a very small effect on EDSS scores. These results have been criticized on the basis that inadequate azathioprine doses were used in some of these trials. Side effects include gastrointestinal, hematological, and hepatic toxicity. Another potential risk of long-term therapy is cancer, although a case-controlled study suggests that short-term use (less than 5 years) is not associated with a significantly increased risk. Careful monitoring of the patient, including blood cell counts and liver function tests, is necessary throughout the course of treatment.

*In the opinion of the Committee, this therapy has been demonstrated to have limited usefulness in selected patients. Although it is generally well tolerated, its use carries risk.*

## Cyclophosphamide

Cyclophosphamide is another immunosuppressive drug that has been used in MS treatment for many years. Its early use was mostly in uncontrolled studies, in which it was often, but not always, reported to improve the condition of patients with chronic progressive MS, especially those with only modest disability at the beginning of treatment. The largest trial performed, a Canadian multicenter study, failed to demonstrate benefit. Cyclophosphamide has many side effects, including hair loss, nausea and vomiting, hemorrhagic cystitis, infertility, and risk of infection. Some clinicians still use cyclophosphamide as a "booster" in rapidly progressive patients, based on reports that it may stabilize the disease. Careful monitoring of the patient, including blood cell counts, liver function tests, and urinalysis, is necessary throughout the course of treatment.

*In the opinion of the Committee, there remains considerable controversy about the merits of this drug in MS in the absence of positive results from large, randomized, and controlled stud-*

*ies. Because its use carries significant risk, further use should be regarded as investigational.*

## Cyclosporin-A

Cyclosporin-A is an effective immunosuppressive agent that is chiefly responsible for improved success rates with kidney, heart, and liver transplants. It also has been found to be effective in some autoimmune diseases. It was studied in a number of clinical trials in MS, the largest involving 547 patients with chronic progressive disease, and was found to slightly reduce the progression rate and delay the time to requiring use of a wheelchair. These marginal to modest benefits from treatment, however, are outweighed by the long-term toxicity of the drug in impairing kidney function and causing hypertension.

> *In the opinion of the Committee, cyclosporin A has some efficacy, but the association with serious side effects makes it an unsuitable therapy in MS.*

## Methotrexate

Methotrexate is another immunosuppressive agent. Low-dose oral administration has been shown to be both effective and relatively nontoxic in other immunologically mediated diseases such as rheumatoid arthritis and psoriasis. An early trial in MS showed some reduction in the relapse rate but no benefit in patients with progressive disease.

In a more recent study, 60 ambulatory patients with progressive MS and moderate to severe disability were treated with methotrexate in a dosage of 7.5 mg weekly or placebo for two years. Patients receiving active treatment showed significantly reduced worsening according to a composite measure of outcome that included the EDSS and tests of arm function, the maximal benefit occurring relatively early in the study. However, the effect of this treatment was not significant when a traditional outcome measure such as the EDSS was used. The effect on MRI activity also was marginal. This low dose of methotrexate was well tolerated, and no patient discontinued treatment because of side effects.

Prolonged use of methotrexate may cause mucosal irritation, gastrointestinal symptoms, hepatotoxicity, pulmonary fibrosis, and bone marrow suppression.

*In the opinion of the Committee, benefit has not been proven, and further studies are needed. Low-dose therapy seems to be well tolerated.*

## Cladribine (2-Chlorodeoxyadenosine)

Cladribine is an immunosuppressive drug that produces a phenomenon of relatively selective lymphocyte killing (apoptosis) because of a resistance of the effects of adenosine deaminase. It was tested in MS patients and has a background in the treatment of lymphoid neoplasms and other autoimmune disorders.

The first-year results of a double-blind, placebo-controlled, crossover study of cladribine in 50 patients with progressive MS, which was designed as a two-year study, were favorable. Neurologic scores and total lesion volumes on MRI were stable or improved in the patients receiving cladribine but continued to deteriorate in patients on placebo. These favorable results could not be replicated in a recent phase III study in which 159 patients with progressive MS were randomized to receive cladribine in two different doses (0.7 or 2.1 mg/kg) or placebo. Patients were assessed monthly for 12 months with serial evaluation of disability scores and semiannual measurement of MRI. Although cladribine treatment had a remarkable effect in reducing the volume of gadolinium enhancement on MRI, a significant effect on disability could not be shown. The side-effect profile of this compound includes bone marrow suppression and increased susceptibility to viral infections (especially herpes zoster).

*In the opinion of the Committee, this therapy has no proven clinical benefit; because its use carries significant risk, it must be considered investigational at this moment.*

## Mitoxantrone

Mitoxantrone is an antineoplastic agent that exerts potent immunomodulatory effects, including suppression of B cell immunity and reduction of T cell numbers. Mitoxantrone shows considerably less acute toxicity than many other anticancer drugs, the most serious side effect being cardiotoxicity. Recently three studies were published in which the effects of this compound were investigated in MS.

A French multicenter study of 42 patients with very active disease compared treatment with either mitoxantrone (20 mg IV monthly) and methylprednisolone (1 g IV monthly) or methylprednisolone alone for six months. Blinded analysis of MRI data showed a significant and very strong suppression of disease activity in favor of the mitoxantrone-treated patients; unblinded clinical assessments also favored the mitoxantrone group.

An Italian study enrolled 51 patients with relapsing-remitting disease in a randomized, placebo-controlled design (8 mg/m$^2$ IV monthly for 1 year) of two years duration. A trend toward reduction in disease activity as measured with clinical and MRI parameters was also found.

More recently, the results of a European multicenter, placebo-controlled, randomized, blinded, phase III study were presented. Patients with secondary progressive MS (n = 194) were randomized to either of two doses of mitoxantrone (5 mg/m$^2$ or 12 mg/m$^2$) or placebo, given intravenously every three months for two years. A significant beneficial effect on relapse rate and disability progression was found in the absence of severe toxicity. MRI data confirmed the beneficial effect on disease activity. Treatment was well tolerated.

When considering treatment with mitoxantrone, it is extremely important that patients with cardiac disease be excluded and that (depending on the dosage regimen used) monthly ECGs, blood counts, and urine samples be taken and six-monthly echocardiographic studies be performed.

*In the opinion of the Committee, present studies suggest that mitoxantrone may be effective in reducing disease activity in MS. Full peer-reviewed publication of the results of the European multicenter study should be awaited before a clear recommendation can be made. The risk of cardiotoxicity at higher cumulative doses is likely to limit the duration of treatment.*

## Sulfasalazine

Sulfasalazine is a well-established and safe drug with known antiinflammatory and immunomodulatory properties; it has been used as a treatment for inflammatory bowel disease for a number of decades. More recently, it also proved to have a favorable impact on rheumatoid arthritis. The results of a large Mayo Clinic–Canadian cooperative, double-blind, placebo-controlled, phase III trial of sulfasalazine in active MS were recently reported. A total of 199 ambulatory MS patients with active disease were treated with sulfasalazine up to 2 grams a day or placebo and were evaluated for a minimum of three years (mean follow-up 3.7 years). Even though the short-term (2-year) response seemed to be favorable, the drug ultimately failed to slow or prevent disability progression as measured by the primary outcome (confirmed worsening of the EDSS score by at least 1 point on two consecutive 3-month visits).

*In the opinion of the Committee, this therapy does not have benefit in MS.*

## Interferon Alpha

Interferon alpha is, like IFN beta, a type 1 IFN (for explanation see section on IFN beta). They both use the same receptor, and therefore it is plausible that IFN alpha might also have a favorable impact on the course of MS.

The first large trial of recombinant IFN alpha studied 98 patients for one year in a double-blind, randomized, placebo-controlled manner, and this trial showed no clear benefit. More recently, a six-month study of 20 patients was done in Italy with MRI monitoring. New or enlarging lesions occurred more often in scans of placebo-treated patients, and IFN alpha–treated patients had fewer exacerbations. The latter study used higher doses of IFN alpha than had been used in earlier trials, given by every-other-day intramuscular injection.

*In the opinion of the Committee, the rationale of this therapy is plausible and the treatment might well be effective, but larger trials are necessary to establish its safety and efficacy.*

## Corticosteroids

Chronic treatment with glucocorticoids has failed to demonstrate a beneficial effect on either the progression of disability or the rate of relapses. In addition, it may induce severe adverse effects, including osteoporosis, aseptic bone necrosis, proximal muscle weakness, hypertension, hyperglycemia, cataracts, and psychiatric events.

*In the opinion of the Committee, chronic therapy with corticosteroids is contraindicated in MS because of lack of efficacy and reported harmful effects (for pulse treatment with steroids see Chapter 2).*

## Interferon Gamma

*In the opinion of the Committee, this therapy is contraindicated in MS because of reported harmful effects (for explanation see section on interferon beta).*

## Plasmapheresis

In a large, multicenter, placebo-controlled, Canadian study, the value of chronic plasmapheresis (PE) could not be proven. In this study, over a two-year period, PE in association with oral cyclophosphamide and prednisone did not prevent progression of MS disability any more than placebo and sham PE.

*In the opinion of the Committee, the rationale behind this therapy is plausible, but it has not been extensively tested so far and therefore must be regarded as experimental.*

## Total Lymphoid Irradiation

Total lymphoid irradiation (TLI), a radical immunosuppressive modality that attempts to destroy most lymphoid tissues, was previously reported to inhibit the progression of MS. However, at least one other study did not confirm these favorable findings. The complications of TLI can be major, including overwhelming infection, pericarditis, secondary cancer, and gonadal dysfunction.

*In the opinion of the Committee, the risks of this treatment are too high to justify the modest benefits reported.*

## Acyclovir (Zovirax®) and Other Antiviral Agents

There still is the possibility that viruses play an important role in the etiopathogenesis of MS. Therefore, a randomized, double-blind study of acyclovir, an agent commonly used for the treatment of herpes simplex infections, was performed. Sixty patients with relapsing-remitting MS were treated with acyclovir 800 mg three times a day or placebo. A 34 percent reduction in the annual relapse rate was reported during active treatment, warranting further research of acyclovir and related agents.

*In the opinion of the Committee, the rationale behind this therapy is partly plausible, but it has not been extensively tested so far and therefore must be regarded as experimental.*

### BONE MARROW TRANSPLANTATION AND HEMOPOIETIC STEM CELL TRANSPLANTATION

Bone marrow transplantation (BMT) is widely used in a number of neoplastic diseases, and more recently there are a number of reports suggesting that it may also be beneficial in several autoimmune diseases. The procedure consists of a severe immunosuppressive regimen provided by high-dose chemotherapy or total body irradiation followed by IV infusion (transplantation) of bone marrow–derived hematopoietic stem cells. During the first months after BMT, transplant recipients are exposed to many sources of complications, some of which are potentially lethal. The procedure has been shown to be effective in EAE, and there are anecdotal (poorly documented) reports of therapeutic efficacy in MS. A European Study Group for Blood and Marrow Transplantation is in the process of developing guidelines to define criteria for patient selection and transplantation procedures for studies to be initiated in the near future.

*In the opinion of the Committee, the rationale of this therapy is plausible and warrants investigation in well-designed studies carried out in centers with experience in managing profoundly immunocompromised patients. BMT carries serious risk.*

## Treatments Under Development

As indicated previously, a growing amount of evidence suggests that a disturbance of immunologic function in which lymphocytes, macrophages, and cytokines play crucial roles is of importance in the pathogenesis of MS. Therefore, a number of interventions have been designed to alter or block various steps that have been recognized as important in the inflammatory and immunologic pathways.

A number of fundamentally different strategies can be identified:

- To develop agents that induce more selective immunosuppression in an attempt to overcome the potential side effects of global immunosuppression.

- To develop compounds that have an effect on cytokine production by shifting the balance from the production of proinflammatory cytokines IL-2, IFN gamma, tumor necrosis factor-alpha (TNF-alpha) to production of antiinflammatory cytokines IL-4, IL-5, and IL-10. The results of the studies(that showed that IFN beta reduces both clinical and MRI signs of disease activity and the subsequent observations that this might well be related to an effect on this balance between the production of pro- and antiinflammatory cytokines)has been a major stimulus for research to be directed to this area. Some experimental evidence, however, suggests that this type of immune deviation may result in enhanced autoantibody production and more severe disease.
- To develop compounds that have an effect on the initiation of the immunologic response in which T lymphocytes are being activated when antigen that is presented by antigen-presenting cells is recognized by specialized receptors on the T lymphocytes. Findings in the animal model EAE have suggested that this approach might be successful.
- To develop compounds that stabilize the blood–brain barrier in such a way that activated immune cells are less likely to be able to enter the CNS. The relevance of this type of mechanism has been emphasized by MRI studies that have been performed on patients who initiated treatment with IFN beta, in which it was demonstrated that part of the efficacy of IFN beta might be related to it.

## Monoclonal Antibodies to (Subsets of) Lymphocytes

Monoclonal antibodies are very specific antibodies that can be very specifically targeted to certain molecules [e.g., on (subsets of) lymphocytes] and thereby represent a way of inducing more selective immunosuppression.

In the United Kingdom, 29 MS patients were treated with IV infusions of a humanized *monoclonal antibody CAMPATH-1H* (antiCDw52). This treatment induced a profound systemic lymphocyte depletion and prevented the occurrence of new lesions on MRI. Remarkably, during longer follow-up a substantial proportion of these patients worsened clinically in the absence of new lesion development; the compound also induced hyperthyroidism in approximately one-third of patients.

A phase II study in which a chimeric *anti-CD4 monoclonal antibody* was applied to induce a reduction in the number of CD4+ lymphocytes did not show an effect of this intervention on the disease activity as measured by MRI.

## Agents That Interfere with Cytokine Production and Activity

Especially in this respect, TNF-alpha has been considered to be of great importance: it is expressed in MS lesions, and there seems to be a correlation between production of TNF-alpha and clinical disease activity. In addition, it has been demonstrated to exert a number of potentially harmful effects, such as stimulating the production of many other proinflammatory cytokines and showing cytotoxicity for oligodendrocytes, the myelin-producing cells of the CNS. On the other hand, TNF-alpha has been documented to be antiinflammatory. Specific biological inhibitors of TNF in the form of *anti-TNF monoclonal antibodies* and *soluble TNF receptor constructs* have become available and have been applied in preliminary studies in MS. In a pilot study, two people with rapidly progressive MS were treated with IV infusions of a humanized monoclonal anti-TNF antibody. A transient increase in the number of active lesions on MRI and a transient increase in cells and immunoglobulin in the CSF, suggestive of immune activation and increase in disease activity related to the treatment, was observed. A North American phase II study of 168 patients, most of whom had relapsing-remitting MS, using a soluble TNF receptor fusion protein (Lenercept®) demonstrated that the number of Lenercept®-treated patients experiencing exacerbations was significantly increased compared with patients receiving placebo. These results underline the necessity to better understand the role of TNF-alpha activity in MS.

## Other Cytokines

Early phase I and II trials are under way to examine the therapeutic potential of antiinflammatory cytokines TGF-beta and IL-10 that have become available as recombinant products. Based on findings that IL-12 production is correlated with disease progression and that EAE can be prevented by antibodies against IL-12, a trial using these antibodies in MS is planned. At this time it is too early to assess the potential role of these treatment modalities in MS. We must be aware of the fact that many cytokines can exert different functions under different conditions and—perhaps of even more importance—mainly have local effects over very short distances, as a consequence of which systemic administration might induce unanticipated effects.

*Pentoxifyllin* is a phosphodiesterase IV inhibitor that has been shown to induce a switch from pro- to antiinflammatory cytokine production and to decrease production of TNF-alpha; it has been shown to be effective in suppressing EAE. Its potential in MS has been investigated in a number of pilot studies. The effects on various immune parameters (in both blood and CSF) and clinical and MRI assessments, however, have been disappointing so far. One study suggests that it can be effectively used as an adjunct to treatment with IFN beta to suppress early side effects associated with this treatment.

## Agents That Induce Specific Immunosuppression

Specific immunosuppression is targeted to interfere with the events that lead to activation of T lymphocytes at the level of the so-called trimolecular complex; disease-relevant antigens are here presented by antigen-presenting cells to T cells expressing the appropriate T cell receptor, resulting in generation of proinflammatory myelin-reactive lymphocytes. This can, for example, be achieved by administrating molecules (e.g., monoclonal antibodies) that inactivate the relevant part of the T cell receptor, by administrating peptide molecules that compete for binding with the T cell receptor, or by T cell vaccination. The concept of interfering at this level, although very attractive in theory, poses several problems, the major one being that an immune deviation specific for MS so far has not been found. Therefore, there is considerable skepticism with regard to the therapeutic potential in MS for this type of intervention, even though it has previously been shown to be very effective in the animal model EAE. Even if an initially very specific T cell–mediated immune response could be identified and targeted, the feasibility of such therapy is diminished because immune responses diversify (epitope spreading) with longer duration.

## Oral Myelin

Following the initial pilot trial of oral tolerization with myelin antigens, a multicenter, randomized, double-blind, placebo-controlled trial of oral myelin has been completed. This phase III pivotal trial was performed at 14 centers in the United States and Canada. More than 500 patients with relapsing-remitting MS (EDSS scores 4.5 or lower) were included and stratified according to sex and DR2 phenotype (because patients who were males or HLA-DR2 negative tended to have a better response in a pilot trial). The primary end point for this two-year study was relapse rate, and secondary end points were MRI-based. Results from this trial do not show any significant advantage of oral myelin (Myloral®) over placebo.

## Administration of Myelin Basic Protein and Other Peptides

A phase I clinical trial has been completed in which the effect of intrathecal and intravenous administration of myelin basic protein (MBP) synthetic peptides on levels of free and bound titers of antimyelin basic protein in CSF was measured. No significant adverse effects were reported. Recently, studies have been initiated that investigate safety and efficacy of peptide analogues of MBP (altered peptide ligands). These peptides are believed to bind to relevant T cell receptors without leading to T cell activation in a way that they rather induce production of antiinflammatory than proinflammatory cytokines. Theoretically, this form of peptide therapy may lead to a treatment that specifically inactivates those T cells implicated in MS.

## T Cell (Receptor) Vaccination

Despite the fact that firm evidence for unique T cell characteristics in MS is lacking up until now, pilot studies have been performed in which patients were vaccinated with irradiated T cells reactive to MBP. The "vaccine" is designed to specifically kill those T cells that are thought to be disease-inducing. Larger clinical trials have recently been started in both the United States and Europe.

## Agents That Reduce Blood–Brain Barrier Injury

This type of intervention comes into play very early in the disease process, when immune cells from the blood stream are forcing their way into the brain and spinal cord through the blood–brain barrier, the tight wall lining blood vessels that normally protects the brain and spinal cord from invasion. Observations in patients treated with IFN beta as well as in animals with EAE have shown that reducing the permeability of the blood–brain barrier can be an effective way to prevent new lesion formation.

Monoclonal antibodies to adhesion molecules, recombinant soluble adhesion molecules that compete with the binding of activated T cells, and other competitive blockers of adhesion molecules such as the selectins are becoming available for future exploratory trials in MS. A small, placebo-controlled, pilot study applying short-term treatment with a monoclonal antibody against the leukocyte integrin receptor $alpha_4beta_1$ (Antegren®) has recently been performed at several centers in the United Kingdom. Seventy-two patients with either relapsing-remitting or secondary progressive MS were enrolled, and MRI showed evidence of short-term efficacy. The long-term effect of this treatment is yet to be investigated.

The process of proteolytic disruption of the extracellular matrix of the blood–brain barrier by so-called matrix-degrading metalloproteinases (MMPs) has received increasing attention in recent years. Recent studies suggest that the beneficial effect of both steroids and IFN beta in MS might be at least partially related to a reduction in the activity of some MMPs and increased production of tissue inhibitors to MMPs. Inhibitors of MMPs have been shown to be effective in suppressing EAE.

Future studies might also include the administration of neuroprotective agents or molecules that would facilitate axonal regrowth, the administration of growth factors that promote the proliferation and survival of oligodendrocytes, the cells that make myelin, and the transplantation of cells (e.g., neural stem cells or progenitor cells) that are capable of making new myelin.

*In the opinion of the Committee, for all approaches mentioned in this section, "Treatments Under Development," more research is needed before their role in the treatment of MS can be determined. At this time their use cannot be recommended outside the context of well-designed clinical trials.*

*Although proof has become available that we have developed the tools to generate intervention strategies that are effective in the treatment of patients with MS, we must be careful that in this atmosphere of optimism we do not too easily adopt new therapeutic approaches on the basis of results of small studies without phase III trials involving large numbers of patients being performed. This has recently been reemphasized by the unfortunate experience with roquinimex (Linomide®), an immunomodulatory agent that had shown promising effects in two phase II studies but had to be withdrawn from phase III studies, which at that time included almost 1,500 patients, because of unexpected serious (cardiovascular) side effects. In a disease such as MS, where disability generally accumulates slowly over many years, severe side effects, even if infrequent, might invalidate a therapeutic approach.*

*Which of the interventions described in this chapter will ultimately be a worthwhile addition to our present therapeutic armamentarium can only be decided on the basis of the results obtained in a clinical development program that incorporates appropriate study designs of sufficient duration and sufficiently high numbers of patients.*

# Guide for Further Reading

## On Interferon Beta

- The IFNB Multiple Sclerosis Study Group. Interferon beta-1b is effective in relapsing remitting multiple sclerosis. I. Clinical results. *Neurology* 1993; 43:655–661.
- Paty DW, Li DKB, the UBC MS/MRI Study Group, and the IFNB Multiple Sclerosis Study Group. Interferon beta-1b is effective in relapsing remitting multiple sclerosis. II. MRI analysis. *Neurology* 1993; 43:662–667.
- Jacobs LD, Cookfair DL, Rudick RA, et al. Intramuscular interferon beta-1a for disease progression in relapsing multiple sclerosis. *Ann Neurol* 1996; 39:285–294.
- Rudick RA, Goodkin DE, Jacobs LD, et al. The impact of interferon beta-1a on neurologic disability in multiple sclerosis. *Neurology* 1997; 49:358–363.
- Simon JH, Jacobs LD, Campion M, et al. Magnetic resonance studies of intramuscular interferon beta-1a for relapsing multiple sclerosis. *Ann Neurol* 1998; 43:79–87.
- PRISMS Study Group. Randomised, double-blind placebo-controlled study of interferon beta-1a in relapsing remitting multiple sclerosis. *Lancet* 1998; 352:1498–1504.
- European Study Group on interferon beta-1b in secondary progressive MS. Placebo-controlled multicentre randomised trial of interferon beta-1b in treatment of secondary progressive multiple sclerosis. *Lancet* 1998; 352:1491–1497.
- Cross AH, Antel JP. Antibodies to beta-interferons in multiple sclerosis. Can we neutralize the controversy? *Neurology* 1998; 50:1206–1208.
- The Once Weekly Interferon for MS Group. Evidence of interferon beta-1a dose response in relapsing remitting MS. The OWIMS study. *Neurology* 1999; 53:679–686.
- Li DKB, Paty DW, UBC MS/MRI Analysis Research Group, and the PRISMS Study Group. Magnetic resonance imaging results of the PRISMS trial: A randomized, double-blind, placebo-controlled study of interferon beta-1a in relapsing remitting multiple sclerosis. *Ann Neurol* 1999; 46:197–206.
- Miller DH, Molyneux PD, Barker GJ, et al. Effect of interferon beta-1b on magnetic resonance imaging outcomes in secondary progressive multiple sclerosis: Results of a European multicenter randomized double-blind placebo-controlled trial. *Ann Neurol* 1999; 46:850–859.

## On Glatiramer Acetate

- Johnson KP, Brooks BR, Cohen JA, et al. Copolymer 1 reduces relapse rate and improves disability in relapsing-remitting multiple sclerosis: Results of a phase III multicenter, double-blind, placebo-controlled trial. *Neurology* 1995; 45:1268–1276.
- Johnson KP, Brooks BR, Cohen JA, et al. Extended use of glatiramer acetate (Copaxone) is well tolerated and maintains its clinical effect on multiple sclerosis relapse rate and degree of disability. *Neurology* 1998; 50:701–708.

## On Intravenous Immunoglobulin

- Fazekas F, Deisenhammer F, Strasser-Fuchs S, et al. Randomized placebo-controlled trial of monthly intravenous immunoglobulin therapy in relapsing remitting multiple sclerosis. *Lancet* 1997; 349:589–593.
- Sorensen PS, Wanscher B, Jensen CV, et al. Intravenous immunoglobulin G reduces MRI activity in relapsing multiple sclerosis. *Neurology* 1998; 50:1273–1281.
- Lisak RP. Intravenous immunoglobulins in multiple sclerosis. *Neurology* 1998; 51(Suppl 5):S25–S29.

## On Azathioprine

- Yudkin PL, Ellison GW, Ghezzi A, et al. Overview of azathioprine treatment in multiple sclerosis. *Lancet* 1991; 338:1051–1055.

## On Cyclophosphamide

- Weiner HL, Mackin GA, Orav EJ, et al. Intermittent cyclophosphamide pulse therapy in progressive multiple sclerosis: Final report of the Northeast Cooperative Multiple Sclerosis Treatment Group. *Neurology* 1993; 43:910–918.
- Noseworthy JH, Ebers GC, Gent M, et al. The Canadian Cooperative trial of cyclophosphamide and plasma exchange in progressive multiple sclerosis. *Lancet* 1991; 337:441–446.

## On Cyclosporin-A

- Multiple Sclerosis Study Group. Efficacy and toxicity of cyclosporine in chronic progressive multiple sclerosis: A randomized, double-blinded, placebo-controlled clinical trial. *Ann Neurol* 1990; 27:591–605.

## On Methotrexate

- Goodkin DE, Rudick RA, VanderBrug Medendorp S, et al. Low-dose (7.5 mg) oral methotrexate reduces the rate of progression in chronic progressive multiple sclerosis. *Ann Neurol* 1995; 37:30–40.

## On Cladribine

- Rice GPA, for the Cladribine Clinical Study Group; and Filippi M and Comi GC, for the Cladribine MRI Study Group. Cladribine and progressive MS: Clinical and MRI outcomes of a multicenter controlled trial. *Neurology* 2000; 54:1145–1155.

## On Mitoxantrone

- Millefiorini E, Gasperini C, Pozzilli C, et al. Randomised placebo-controlled trial of mitoxantrone in relapsing-remitting multiple sclerosis: A 24-month clinical and MRI outcome. *J Neurol* 1997; 244:153–159.

■ Edan G, Miller D, Clanet M, et al. Therapeutic effect of mitoxantrone combined with methylprednisolone in multiple sclerosis: A randomised multicentre study of active disease using MRI and clinical criteria. *J Neurol Neurosurg Psychiatry* 1997; 62:112–118.

## On Sulfasalazine

■ Noseworthy JH, O'Brien P, Erickson BJ, et al. The Mayo Clinic–Canadian Cooperative trial of sulfasalazine in active multiple sclerosis. *Neurology* 1998; 51:1342–1352.

## On Plasmapheresis

■ Weinshenker BG, O'Brien PC, Petterson TM, et al. A randomized trial of plasma exchange in acute central nervous system inflammatory demyelinating disease. *Ann Neurol* 1999; 46:878–886.

## On Acyclovir

■ Lycke J, Svennerholm B, Hjelmquist E, et al. Acyclovir treatment of relapsing remitting multiple sclerosis. A randomized, placebo-controlled, double-blind study. *J Neurol* 1996; 243:214–224.

## On Treatments Under Development

■ Hohlfeld R. Biotechnological agents in the immunotherapy of multiple sclerosis. *Brain* 1997; 120:865–916.

# CHAPTER 4

# Symptomatic Treatment and Rehabilitation

Multiple sclerosis (MS) involves multiple areas of the central nervous system (CNS) and therefore can produce a diverse range of symptoms, from visual loss to pain, fatigue, and paraparesis (Table 4-1). In the initial stages of the condition, the symptoms are often isolated or, if multiple, relate to a single area of inflammation, although multiple areas may be involved (e.g., optic nerve and spinal cord). Symptoms usually are transient; even in these early stages recovery may be less than complete, leaving residual disturbance, or symptoms may reemerge with exercise (e.g., Uhthoff's phenomenon). There are some people in whom the initial presentation, which usually is a mild spastic paraparesis (spasticity and weakness that leads to difficulty in walking), progressively worsens without any remission (primary progressive MS).

In time, the majority of patients develop an increasing range of symptoms, many of which worsen slowly, resulting in progressive and complex disability. This poses particular problems in terms of management in that the symptoms tend to interact with each other and it may be inappropriate to treat one symptom in isolation. For example, the carrying out of clean, intermittent self-catheterization to manage bladder emptying must take into account the patient's cognitive ability, upper limb dexterity, and lower limb mobility (in relation to spasticity, etc.). It is also important to appreciate that the treatment of one symptom may worsen another, such as the effects of

Table 4-1 Symptoms in Multiple Sclerosis

Cognitive dysfunction
Fatigue, temperature lability
Visual disturbance
Speech/swallowing disturbance
Poor dexterity—weakness, tremor, sensory disturbance
Bladder/bowel/sexual dysfunction
Poor mobility—weakness, spasticity, ataxia
Pain

antispasticity or antidepressant agents in people already suffering from severe fatigue. This is, at least in part, the rationale behind the need for goal-orientated multidisciplinary rehabilitation at this stage of the condition.

This chapter discusses the treatment of individual symptoms followed by rehabilitation and service provision. In contrast to the previous section, which was able to call upon evidence from randomized control trials, there is a paucity of such data available in symptomatic management and rehabilitation. Where studies have been carried out, they tended to be small and poorly designed. To address this deficit, two important initiatives have taken place over the last two years—the setting up of the Multiple Sclerosis Council for Clinical Practice Guidelines (MSCCPG) and the establishment of the Cochrane Collaboration for Multiple Sclerosis.

The MSCCPG is a collaboration of a number of key organizations involved in MS, including the Consortium of Multiple Sclerosis Societies (North America), Rehabilitation in Multiple Sclerosis (RIMS—European Organization of MS Centres), and the International Federation of Multiple Sclerosis Societies (IFMSS). The MSCCPG has published guidelines on fatigue and bladder management and has just completed guidelines on spasticity. The Cochrane Collaboration is applying the principle of evaluating randomized controlled trials to look at aspects of the management of MS. In relation to symptomatic management, current protocols include the role of the aminopyridines in MS, the treatment of spasticity, and the evaluation of rehabilitation.

## Symptomatic Treatment of MS

The treatment of individual symptoms is discussed in this section, bearing in mind that the majority of people have multiple symptoms that interact in a complex and disabling fashion. For example, poor mobility may result from any or all of the following: lower limb and truncal weakness, spasticity, cerebellar ataxia, reduced sensory input, or reduced and/or distorted vision. Similarly, fatigue, mood disturbance, and cognitive dysfunction also interact and may complicate both evaluation and subsequent management. Even when considering individual symptoms, it is essential to appreciate that drug treatment is of limited value but often is optimally used in association with therapy. For example, spasticity can only rarely be managed by oral antispasticity agents alone, but it may be greatly helped by a combination of physical therapy and medication. A further important component is the recently highlighted role of patient education. This is particularly important in the management of symptoms such as spasticity, where basic practical issues such as posture, standing program, and so forth are crucial, but patient education applies equally to most, if not all, other symptoms such as ataxia and fatigue.

## Spasticity

Spasticity is a frequent symptom in MS and is seen to a greater or lesser extent in up to 75 percent of patients. It is a complex, poorly understood symptom that is just one component of the upper motor neuron syndrome. In MS the lower limbs are more markedly affected by spasticity than the arms. Spasticity may be associated with pain, painful extensor and flexor spasms, clonus, and underlying weakness. Extensor spasticity of the legs, particularly of the quadriceps, might be considered advantageous for standing, walking, and transferring. However, sudden loss of tone may also occur when the muscle reaches a certain crucial length as a result of increasing resistance and progressive stretching. Spasticity is associated with structural changes in the muscles (thixotrophy) leading to further resistance to movement and shortening. Functionally, spasticity can reduce mobility and dexterity, while spasms may prevent transfers, hinder comfortable sitting and lying posture, and affect sleep.

The treatment of spasticity should not be aimed at its removal per se but rather at improving function, easing care, or alleviating pain. Key components in the management of spasticity include patient education, physiotherapy input, and the judicious use of drug treatment. This should include awareness that noxious stimuli, such as urinary tract infections, bowel impaction, and ingrown toenails, may worsen spasticity and should emphasize the importance of correct positioning in lying and sitting and the value of a standing program. Treatment may be divided into oral therapy, drugs given by other routes (intrathecal, intraneural, or intramuscular), and surgery. It must be remembered that whatever treatment is chosen, expert monitoring is required. Furthermore, MS-related spasticity tends to change over time, and it is important to reevaluate treatments at regular intervals.

There are few trials of antispasticity agents in MS, and those that exist usually are of small numbers where the pattern of spasticity is inadequately described, the objectives of treatment are not specified, and only short- to medium-term outcomes are assessed. In clinical practice it is suggested that only one substance be used at a time, although there may be a rationale for combining drugs if a single agent is ineffective or only partially effective. Of the available agents, baclofen has undergone most evaluation, of both the oral and intrathecal routes, and tizanidine has been the most recently licensed drug in the United Kingdom and the United States. Most of the studies were carried out 20 to 30 years ago, and many focused on spinal cord injury. The management of severe spasticity may be best provided by a multidisciplinary clinic that incorporates neurologic, physiologic, and physiotherapy expertise and can provide a wide range of treatment options.

### ORAL AGENTS

**Baclofen**   This γ-aminobutyric acid (GABA)-B receptor agonist acts mainly on the presynaptic and postsynaptic terminals of primary fibers of the spinal cord both to reduce the release of amino acids and to antagonize their actions. It is particularly useful in the treatment of painful spasms and increased tone of spinal origin, although functional benefits have been more difficult to demonstrate. In a large study of 759 patients with MS, 70 percent showed marked improvement in spasticity (defined as a two-step reduction on the Ashworth Scale) and flexor spasms. A beneficial effect on spasms and hypertonicity was also seen in a small, double-blind, placebo-controlled, cross-over study that involved 22 patients, 11 of whom had MS. The efficacy of baclofen has been shown to be equal to, if not greater than, that of diazepam. Baclofen is given three times a day in doses starting at 5 to 10 mg in stepwise increases until the desired effect is achieved and/or side effects such as drowsiness, fatigue, and muscle weakness become unacceptable, usually reaching a dose of between 60 and 80 mg a day. Side effects are reported to affect up to 45 percent of patients. Abrupt discontinuation may result in severe withdrawal symptoms, which include hallucinations and seizures.

**Tizanidine**   This imidazoline derivative, which is closely related to clonidine, acts by stimulating $\beta 2$-adrenergic receptors in the spinal cord. A number of studies have suggested that its efficacy is similar to that of baclofen, and more recently it was evaluated in two double-blind, placebo-controlled trials in the United Kingdom and the United States involving 187 and 220 patients, respectively. In the American trial, tizanidine reduced spasms and clonus significantly but had no effect on spasticity as measured on the Ashworth Scale, and although the patients rated the drug significantly better on efficacy, the assessing physician did not. In the U.K. trial, a 20 percent reduction in spasticity was reported, and 75 percent of patients receiving the drug reported a subjective benefit without an increase in muscle weakness. However, no improvement in mobility-related activities of daily living was found. The suggestion that it may not cause weakness is of therapeutic value. It is suggested that it be started at a low dose, 2 mg three times a day, and gradually increased up to a maximum of between 18 and 36 mgs. A long-acting preparation that may be taken once daily is available in some countries. The most frequent side effects are tiredness, drowsiness, and dry mouth. Liver function tests must be checked before and after treatment because transient hepatotoxicity may occur.

**Dantrolene and Benzodiazepines**   Few studies have evaluated the role of these drugs or compared their efficacy in the management of spasticity. However, because dantrolene has a peripheral target of action and exerts its effect within the muscle itself by inhibiting the release of calcium ions from the sarcoplasmic reticulum, thereby preventing muscle contraction, it is theoretically a useful additional agent if centrally acting drugs are not effective. It is thought to be more effective in treating spasms and clonus than hypertonicity, and long-term benefit has been documented. However, it is poorly tolerated, with side effects including drowsiness, weakness, and fatigue, and occasionally hepatotoxicity, which may be irreversible.

Benzodiazepines have three potential antispasticity actions: suppression of sensory impulses from muscle and skin receptors, potentiation of GABA action postsynaptically, and inhibition of excitatory descending pathways. The efficacy of diazepam has been evaluated in a small, double-blind, cross-over trial of 21 patients with spastic paraparesis. It may be used as additional therapy in resistant cases of spasticity. Its role is limited by side effects, including drowsiness and dependence.

**Other Oral Agents**   A range of drugs has been tried in MS-related spasticity, and reports involving small numbers have appeared in the literature. These drugs include clonazepam, memantine, glycine, L-threonine, vigabatrin, and, more recently, gabapentin. There is increasing pressure to evaluate the role of cannabinoids in spasticity and MS, and a major study has commenced in the United Kingdom.

OTHER ROUTES

In very severe spasticity, high doses of oral agents are likely to be either ineffective or not tolerated, and drugs may best be given intrathecally via a subcutaneously placed infusion pump. Although this may be considered an invasive treatment, it is very efficient, and less than one hundredth of the oral dose is required to achieve the required effect. The intrathecal route was originally described by Kelly and Gautier-Smith for the use of phenol, but more recently it has been evaluated by Penn for baclofen. Dramatic effects on both tone, as measured by the Ashworth Scale, and spasm frequency were seen in MS and spinal cord injury. Some effect on function, particularly relating to transfers and self-care, has also been reported, but few investigators have evaluated a potential effect on quality of life. In this treatment, the effect is initially tested by bolus injection of 25 to 100 mg given via a lumbar puncture before considering continuous drug application through an electronically programmed drug delivery system. Long-term treatment using intrathecal baclofen (ITB) has been evaluated and found to be beneficial. The main complications are technical and include pump malfunction, catheter-related problems (kinking, breaking, displacement), local inflammation, and, rarely, spinal meningitis. Although the original studies were restricted to patients who were wheelchair users, ITB is now being used with encouraging results in more ambulatory patients. It should be used as part of a goal-orientated rehabilitation program, and careful assessment and selection is essential.

There has been a recent resurgence in interest in intrathecal phenol (4 mg or 2.5 mg in glycerine), which may be useful in improving care and posture in severely disabled patients who no longer have bowel and bladder function and in whom sensation in the lower limbs is absent. In a recent retrospective study of 21 patients, 16 of whom had MS, benefit was seen in all patients, which translated into functional gains in most. Local treatment, with either nerve route injection with phenol and other agents or muscle injection with botulinum toxin, is also used, although again there are few studies available for their evaluation. A recent double-blind, placebo-controlled, dose ranging study evaluated the role of botulinum toxin (Dysport 500, 1000, 1500 units) in 74 MS patients with severe adductor spasticity. Range of hip movement and tone were improved in the treated groups, but all four groups had reduced spasms, showing improvement on a global rating scale. Only the 1000 and 1500 unit groups had improved hygiene scores, and the latter had the highest incidence of side effects. In general, however, botulinum toxin is considered to be more useful in the treatment of distal muscles in the arms and legs, and most practitioners are discouraged by the frequent large doses required for proximal lower limb spasticity in MS.

Although a range of neurosurgical procedures is available in the management of spasticity, none have gained acceptance in the context of MS. There are relatively few data available to evaluate potential benefit.

*In the view of the Committee, spasticity remains a very disabling symptom that often is poorly managed. There is a range of treatment options that have a moderate evidence base. However, a coordinated approach to management is essential, and there is a need for more effective oral agents with a better side-effect profile.*

## Ataxia

Ataxia may be defined as a lack of or reduction in coordination and is invariably associated with tremor (i.e., an involuntary, rhythmic, oscillatory movement of a body part). These symptoms occur in 75 percent of patients with MS and most frequently manifest as upper limb intention tremor. They are both severely disabling and embarrassing, affecting upper limb function, gait, and, in severe cases, standing and sitting balance. The tremor of MS is frequently only one component of a complex movement disorder that includes dysmetria and other ataxic features, and the underlying mechanisms are poorly understood. Although inflammatory demyelination in different parts of the cerebellum and related areas may produce a distinct tremor, it is nonetheless extremely difficult to classify individual tremors in patients. It remains one of the most difficult symptoms to manage and is associated with a poor outcome in rehabilitation.

As with spasticity, there are practical components to the management of ataxia, which must be considered before other interventions. These include patient education, improving posture and proximal stability during activities, and the provision of equipment. Weights have not proved to be very successful, although they may be slightly more effective if a computer damping device is incorporated, and a small exploratory study of therapy input suggested modest benefit. Other treatments may be divided into drug therapy, which is limited and often not well tolerated, and more invasive surgical intervention, including thalamotomy and thalamic stimulation.

## MEDICAL TREATMENT

Few drugs have been evaluated and none adequately. Isoniazid (with pyridoxine) has been shown to be of limited benefit in a number of small studies. It showed some effect in 10 of 13 patients, although this did not translate into improved function, while four of six patients in a second study showed sufficient benefit that they wished to continue the drug. It is thought to be more useful in postural tremor with an intention component than in pure intention tremor. Up to 1200 mg a day in divided doses has been used, increasing gradually from 200 mg twice a day. This drug, which was the first to undergo a randomized control trial for the treatment of MS, is not well tolerated and causes gastrointestinal disturbance.

There has been even less evaluation of other drugs, including carbamazepine, clonazepam, and buspirone. Ethyl alcohol and propranolol have not been found to be useful. Although a single-blind, cross-sectional study evaluating the role of carbamazepine in cerebellar tremor in 10 patients (7 with MS) suggested some benefit, it has also been suggested that this agent worsened ataxia. More recently, the 5-HT3 antagonist ondansetron has been evaluated, given by both intravenous (IV) and oral routes. Although the IV studies looked promising, the more recent placebo-controlled, double-blind, parallel-group study was negative. Fifty-two patients, the majority of whom had MS, were randomized, and the treatment arm received 8 mg per day for one week. Although some benefit in the nine-hole peg test was seen in the treated arm, there was no difference between the groups on a global ataxia rating scale.

## SURGICAL INTERVENTION

Although thalamotomy of the ventral intermediate nucleus (VIN) has been shown to be beneficial in the tremor of Parkinson's disease, there has been limited evaluation of its role in tremor relating to MS. In general, it is not considered to be as effective in this condition. In selected patients with MS, thalamotomy has been reported to alleviate contralateral limb tremor, initially in approximately 65 to 96 percent of cases, although in about 20 percent tremor returns within 12 months.

Functional improvement is estimated to occur in 25 to 75 percent of patients. However, these results are not based on controlled studies, and no prospective study has evaluated the influence of this procedure on overall disability, handicap, and quality of life; side effects have not been adequately quantified, although they may occur in up to 45 percent of patients. Serious side effects, which include hemiparesis, dysphasia, and dysphagia, occur in up to 10 percent of patients. Experience suggests that optimum results are obtained in patients with relatively stable disease, good mobility, and minimal overall disability status—an extremely small group.

Three recent papers have suggested that thalamic stimulation can also alleviate tremor in up to 69 percent of patients in studies involving 13, 5, and 15 patients, respectively. Patients were carefully selected; for example, in one study the five patients reported were from an initial group of 17 patients, and no control study has yet been carried out. Serious side effects may occur. In one recent study comparing thalamic stimulation with lesioning, it is suggested that stimulation is associated with fewer side effects. Other approaches, including extracranial application of brief AC-pulsed electromagnetic fields, dynamic systems with multidegree of freedom orthoses, and robotic arms based on virtual reality, have not been adequately evaluated.

*In the view of the Committee, ataxia and associated tremor are among the most resistant and disabling symptoms to manage. Current strategies are not evidence-based and are of limited benefit.*

## Fatigue

Fatigue, which may be defined as an overwhelming sense of tiredness, lack of energy, and feelings of exhaustion in excess of what might be expected for the associated level of activity, is thought to be the most common and among the most disabling symptoms in MS. Fatigue must be distinguished from depression, although not infrequently these two entities coexist and aggravate each other. Practical issues such as a poor sleep pattern resulting from painful spasms or nocturia also need to be considered. Attempts have been made to distinguish the different types of fatigue in MS, for example, that which follows activity, chronic fatigue, and fatigue associated with a clinical relapse. The underlying mechanisms remain unclear. A range of measures from generic to disease-specific are currently available to evaluate this difficult symptom, some of which are shown in Table 4-2.

Fatigue management programs are the mainstay in the management of this symptom—identifying fatigue as a relevant and disabling symptom and examining daily routine to determine how best to minimize its impact, including energy conservation and work simplification techniques. A graded exercise program has been advocated, although there are limited data to support its usefulness. A study that evaluated the role of aerobic exercise, while showing benefit in maximum aerobic capacity and isometric muscle strength, did not show an effect on fatigue as measured by the Fatigue Impact Scale.

MEDICATION

Two oral agents, amantadine, an antiviral agent that also has antiparkinsonian effects, and pemoline, a CNS stimulant, have been studied in the management of fatigue. A small, cross-over, randomized, control trial of amantadine showed that it had a significant effect on fatigue in relation to placebo. In contrast, a small, randomized, cross-over trial of 40 patients comparing pemoline and placebo showed no significant effect from pemoline, which was poorly tolerated in 25 percent of patients. In the most comprehensive study to date, pemoline and amantadine were compared with placebo. The placebo group received advice on fatigue management. A range of outcome measures, including the generic Fatigue Severity Scale and the six-item MS-Specific Fatigue Scale, were used.

Amantadine showed a benefit over placebo in the MS-Specific Fatigue Scale but not the Fatigue Severity Scale. No benefit was seen with pemoline. On the basis of this study, the authors suggest that amantadine should be the first-line medication for use in MS-related fatigue, although they did caution that a placebo response from either agent is a strong possibility.

Another agent that holds some promise, although it has has never been comprehensively evaluated in fatigue, is the potassium channel blocker 4-aminopyridine. This drug was comprehensively evaluated in a randomized, placebo-controlled, double-blind, cross-over study involving 70 patients with MS. A significant effect on the Expanded Disability Status Scale (EDSS) was seen in the treated group, although side effects, which included paresthesias, dizziness, and gait instability, were common. Longer follow-up has suggested that it may be particularly useful in

Figure 4-2   Levels of Measurement and Examples of Generic and MS-Specific Measures

| Term | Definition | Outcome Measures | |
|---|---|---|---|
| | | Generic | MS-Specific |
| Impairment | Clinical signs/symptoms resulting from nervous system damage | | Functional systems of EDSS Composite measure (US Task Force) |
| Disability | Limitations on activities of daily living from neurologic impairment | Barthel Index (BI) Functional Independence Measure (FIM) Functional Independence Measure/ Functional Assessment Measure (FIM/FAM) | Guy's Neurological Disability Scale (GNDS) Incapacity Status Scale |
| Handicap | Social and environmental consequences from impairment and disability | London Handicap Scale (LHS) | Environmental Status Scale (ESS) |
| Health-related quality of life (QoL) | The satisfaction that people have with health-related dimensions of life, from their own perspective | Short Form-36 (SF-36) Nottingham Health Profile Sickness Impact Profile | MSQoL54 Functional Assessment of MS QoL Instrument (FAMS) MS QoL Inventory (MSQLI) |
| Emotional well-being | | General Health Questionnaire | |
| Symptoms, e.g., fatigue | Overwhelming sense of tiredness or exhaustion in excess of what might be expected from level of activity | Fatigue Impact Scale Fatigue Severity Scale | MS-Specific Fatigue Scale |

fatigue, although the occasional occurrence of an epileptic seizure (usually associated with high levels) remains a concern. A number of small studies of 3-4 diaminopyridine have also suggested some potential benefit. Recent studies of 4-AP have suggested that, given the low dose used clinically, its therapeutic effect may relate to potentiation of synaptic transmission and an increase in skeletal muscle twitch tension rather than the restoration of conduction in demyelinated axons. More recently, encouraging results have been reported from the use of modafinil (Provigil®). A comprehensive strategy is contained within the evidence-based guidelines on fatigue management produced by the MSCCPG.

> *In the view of the Committee, fatigue remains one of the most disabling symptoms in MS, and drug therapy plays a relatively minor role in comparison to more practical approaches to its management.*

## Bladder Dysfunction

Bladder problems are among the most disabling and distressing symptoms in MS. Studies of large groups of patients have suggested that bladder dysfunction occurs in at least 70 percent of those with MS, which perhaps is not surprising when we consider that bladder function is regulated at three interconnected levels of the CNS: the frontal lobes, the pontine micturition center, and the sacral micturition center. Bladder dysfunction in MS usually, although not invariably, results from spinal cord disease and is therefore often associated with sexual dysfunction and pyramidal symptoms such as weakness and spasticity. Urinary urgency and frequency are the most common symptoms, although hesitancy and nocturia may also be problematic. The underlying problems have been described as difficulty with storage and emptying, the former resulting from detrusor hyperreflexia and the latter from detrusor-sphincter dyssynergia.

The management of bladder dysfunction in MS includes two key components, the use of clean intermittent self-catheterization (CISC) to manage incomplete emptying and anticholinergic agents such as oxybutynin to reduce the hyperreflexia that results in inadequate storage. However, because oxybutynin may decrease bladder emptying and therefore increase residual volume, it is important to check the residual before embarking on treatment.

CISC, which was initially introduced in the management of spinal injury, usually is taught by an experienced continence advisor but does depend on the patient's learning a consistently clean technique. Problems may arise if there is severe cognitive impairment. There also are potential practical difficulties if hand function is affected by weakness or tremor or if there is severe adductor spasticity or spasm. Some patients are unhappy about carrying out CISC, and a suprapubic vibrator is a possible alternative for those who are ambulatory. This hand-held, battery-operated device has been shown to reduce the residual volume in 80 percent of ambulant patients.

Only when adequate bladder emptying is achieved can drug treatment for detrusor hyperreflexia be initiated. The anticholinergic agent oxybutynin is the first-line treatment and has been shown to be more effective than propantheline in a small randomized trial involving 34 patients. It usually is commenced at 2.5 mg twice daily, but even this dose may cause dry mouth. The maximum recommended dose is 5 mg three times daily. A long-acting preparation that is taken once daily is available in some countries. Of the other anticholinergic drugs, tolterodine tartrate is a useful alternative to oxybutynin and is given in a dose of 2 mg twice a day. Occasionally, adding imipramine to oxybutynin may be helpful.

If oxybutynin is not helpful or inappropriate, desmopressin may be considered, particularly for nocturia. This synthetic antidiuretic hormone is administered by nasal spray. Several cross-over studies involving relatively small numbers of patients (17 and 22, respectively) have shown that one to two puffs (10–20 µg) at bedtime or during the day can reduce urine output for six to eight hours. Benefit over a prolonged period of time has been described recently in a cohort of 19 patients. The expected side effect of hyponatremia is rarely symptomatic, although headache or malaise should be taken as a warning sign, and extreme caution should be exercised in the over-65 age group, who are more likely to become symptomatic. Wheelchair-bound patients with dependent edema are also at risk of developing water retention because their nocturnal frequency may simply be an indication of resorption of edematous fluid. Desmopressin must never be taken more than once every 24 hours.

In more severe disease, interruption of the spinal pathways leads to the emergence of a new reflex at the sacral level mediated by unmyelinated C fibers that stimulate the detrusor, without the control of the normal inhibitory spinal fibers. This detrusor hyperreflexia may be reduced by the neurotoxic effects of capsaicin on the C fibers, and in a small study an instillation of 1 or 2 mmol of capsaicin dissolved in alcohol has shown a beneficial effect lasting up to five months. Repeated instillations may be required and do not appear to be responsible for any long-term side effects. The potential benefits of an ultrapotent capsinoid substance, resiniferotoxin, are currently being evaluated, as are the effects of a sublingual cannabis preparation.

Biofeedback has also been evaluated in a small study of 20 MS patients, which has suggested some benefit. Pelvic floor rehabilitation combined with electrostimulation was evaluated in an open, controlled, randomized study of two parallel groups with 25 women and 15 men in each group. The treatment arm underwent six sessions of electrostimulation of the pelvic floor muscles followed by regular pelvic floor exercises for six months. Symptoms of urinary urgency, frequency, and incontinence were significantly reduced in the treated group, and this was particularly striking in the male patients.

Permanent catheterization may be necessary in many patients with severe disease as medical treatments become ineffective or impractical. A long-term urethral catheter is rarely advisable because it is likely to be extruded and destroy the bladder neck mechanism. The preferred alternative is a suprapubic catheter, which should be inserted by a urological surgeon and subsequently changed every two months.

> *In the view of the Committee, bladder symptoms usually are amenable to management, often with a combination of self-catheterization and an anticholinergic agent.*

## Bowel Dysfunction

Up to two-thirds of all people with MS complain of bowel dysfunction, frequently in combination with bladder problems. The most common symptoms are constipation and fecal incontinence, which frequently coexist. Understanding of the underlying pathophysiologic mechanisms is limited, and little, if any, evaluation of management strategies has taken place. Possible mechanisms resulting in constipation include slow colonic transit time, abnormal rectal function, and intussusception, while incontinence may result from absent or decreased sensation of rectal filling, poor voluntary contraction of the anal sphincter–pelvic floor, or reduced rectal compliance. Factors unrelated to MS such as obstetric injury to the anal sphincters may also play a role. There are no published studies on the effect of medication on bowel symptoms in MS. Most patients try laxatives and enemas before reporting constipation. Increased dietary fiber or bulk laxatives such as lactulose may be helpful in mild constipation but are unlikely to be of benefit for severe symptoms. Stimulant or osmotic laxatives such as senna and bisacodyl may be useful. Establishing a bowel program is often advocated, although without supportive evidence.

When symptoms of fecal incontinence are mild, infrequent, and not due to impaction with overflow, treatment with loperamide or codeine phosphate may be effective, although these agents must be used with caution if incontinence coexists with constipation. An enema given in the morning may reduce the risk of incontinence during the day.

Evidence-based guidelines have recently been published by the MSCCPG and form the basis for much, although not all, of the content of this section.

*In the view of the Committee, bowel dysfunction in patients with MS remains difficult to manage, with little evidence-based guidance.*

## Sexual Dysfunction

Sexual dysfunction is a common and very distressing symptom that affects up to 70 percent of men and women with MS. It is now discussed more openly and constructively than in the past. There has been an increase in understanding the mechanisms responsible for the symptoms and advances in treatment, although mainly in erectile dysfunction in men. Apart from specific neurologic damage, the development of disability may have a major effect on patients' self-image, which may in turn affect both their relationships and sexual function.

### MANAGEMENT OF SEXUAL DYSFUNCTION IN WOMEN

The most frequently described symptoms include decreased sexual desire, diminished orgasm, difficulties with vaginal lubrication, and fatigue that interferes with sexual activity. Decreased vaginal lubrication can be treated with water-soluble lubricants, and dysesthesias may be relieved with carbamazepine or phenytoin. However, nitrergic nerves are also present in the corpus cavernosum of the clitoris and vaginal wall, so there is good rationale for expecting sildenafil (Viagra®) to have a beneficial effect. A randomized control trial is currently under way.

### MANAGEMENT OF SEXUAL DYSFUNCTION IN MEN

Erectile difficulties are present in between 60 and 80 percent of men with MS, with symptoms ranging from difficulty sustaining an erection for intercourse, with normal nocturnal erections and on waking, to total failure of erectile function and difficulty with ejaculation in more severe disease. Clinical and neurophysiologic evidence strongly suggests a spinal origin of the symptom. Up to 96 percent of patients have pyramidal tract signs, while abnormalities of both tibial and pudendal somatosensory evoked potentials and urodynamically proven hyperreflexia (established as being of spinal origin) are seen in 73 percent and 85 percent, respectively.

The value of discussing and providing relevant information cannot be underestimated. Recent advances in drug treatment, notably sildenafil (Viagra®), which has superseded all previously available therapy, are likely to have a major effect on the impact of this symptom. Release of nitric oxide from nerves supplying the arterioles of the corpora cavernosa increases intracellular levels of cyclic GMP, which results in smooth muscle relaxation and penile erection. The effect of cGMP is terminated by the enzyme phosphodiesterase, and sildenafil is an orally active inhibitor of this enzyme. A double-blind, randomized, placebo-controlled trial of 217 men with clinically definite MS with disability ranging between 2.0 and 6.0 on the EDSS has recently been reported. The study was carried out over 16 weeks and included a four-week run-in period. Patients were randomized to either placebo or 50 mg sildenafil to be taken one hour before intercourse at a maximum of once per day. The dose could be altered to either 100 mg or 25 mg, depending on therapeutic response and tolerability. The primary outcome measure was the International Index of Erectile Function (IIEF). One hundred and two of the 104 patients (98%) in the active arm completed treatment compared with 88 of the 113 patients (77%) receiving placebo.

The ability to achieve and maintain erections was significantly improved in the treatment group compared with controls ($p < 0.0001$), and in those patients with improved erections (sildenafil responders) 92 percent reported an improvement in the ability to have satisfactory sexual activity. Adverse events were predominantly mild in nature, with headache (23.1% active group vs. 5.3% in the placebo arm) and flushing (13.5% vs. 1.8%) being the most common. There were three serious adverse events in each arm, none of which were thought to relate to the treatment. No cardiac symptoms were experienced in the treatment arm, although one patient in the placebo arm had a myocardial infarction during the study. A beneficial effect on related aspects of quality of life was also detected using the Life Satisfaction Checklist and the Erection

Distress Scale. The treated group showed significant benefit in five of the eight components of the checklist, including life as a whole ($p < 0.001$) and sexual life ($p < 0.001$), but also partnership relation ($p < 0.001$), family life ($p < 0.003$), and social contacts ($p < 0.03$).

Intracorporeal pharmacotherapy has been in existence for almost two decades, initially with papaverine but more recently with prostaglandin E1 (alprostadil) at a dose of 20 µg. The latter is rapidly metabolized so that priapism and local fibrosis are very rare. Studies have shown it to be highly efficacious, with few, if any, systemic side effects. However, the disadvantages of having to inject are obvious, and patients frequently report penile pain with this treatment. A recent development for which there is some evidence of efficacy is MUSE®, a medicated urethral system for erection that delivers a pellet of alprostadil into the urethra via a small applicator.

A mixture of nitric oxide–releasing dilatory creams has been evaluated in a placebo-controlled, cross-over study and was beneficial in 58 percent of men, while only 8 percent responded to the placebo. Vacuum pumps are occasionally used but have never been evaluated, and prosthetic surgery is not recommended in patients with MS. The only available agent that is claimed to improve ejaculatory function is yohimbine, which is thought to be an alpha-sympathetic agonist but has never been subjected to rigorous evaluation.

*In the view of the Committee, sexual dysfunction in men, particularly difficulty maintaining an erection, is now treated relatively easily. However, sexual dysfunction in women remains difficult to manage.*

## Pain

Pain is another common symptom in MS and occurs in over 50 percent of patients, with considerable impact on their quality of life. The pain is acute and usually paroxysmal in 15 percent of patients, while in the vast majority of patients it is chronic. Rarely, it may be the presenting symptom. Trigeminal neuralgia is the most common type of acute pain and occurs 300 times more frequently in the MS population than in patients without MS. Lhermitte's symptom and painful tonic spasm may also be included in this category. Chronic pain consists mainly of low back pain resulting from proximal weakness and abnormal posture and gait, pain associated with spasticity, and spasm and dysesthetic extremity pain.

Carbamazepine is the mainstay of treatment of trigeminal neuralgia, whether MS-related or not. If this drug is ineffective or poorly tolerated, there is some evidence to suggest that other anticonvulsants may be useful, particularly phenytoin. More recently, a small study of misoprostol, a prostaglandin E1 analogue, involving seven patients who responded poorly to carbamazepine, has been reported. Five patients showed an immediate and sustained benefit. Gabapentin and lamotrigine also have been reported to be of some benefit. Pain becomes chronic in a small proportion of patients, and surgical intervention may be required in this group, particularly if drug therapy is less than adequate or poorly tolerated. Percutaneous procedures have shown benefit, although reinjection may be necessary. This approach has not been rigorously evaluated. Logically, microvascular decompression should not have a role, although a recent study has suggested benefit in 5 of 10 cases of MS. It should, however, be noted that none of the patients had evidence of a demyelinating plaque in the trigeminal root entry zone, pontine tract, or nuclei.

Chronic pain is more difficult to treat, although there is some evidence to support the use of amitriptyline in dysesthetic pain, followed by carbamazepine, clonazepam, and other anticonvulsant drugs. Physiotherapy to improve proximal stability and incorporate education on improved posture in standing and sitting is the cornerstone of treatment for low back pain. Nonsteroidal antiinflammatory drugs, transcutaneous electrical nerve stimulation (TENS), and a heating pad may all play a useful subsidiary role. Spasticity and spasms may be treated as outlined previously, with attention being paid to their potential to worsen truncal weakness, which may be counterproductive.

> *In the view of the Committee, acute paroxysmal pain usually responds to carbamazepine, and other drugs are also available. Chronic pain is more difficult to manage and is often undertreated. It frequently requires multidisciplinary input and, if severe, may benefit from the expertise of a pain clinic.*

## Other Paroxysmal Symptoms

Although relatively uncommon, other paroxysmal symptoms are highly characteristic of MS and include paroxysmal dysarthria and ataxia, tonic spasms, and paroxysmal sensory symptoms. These symptoms are thought to relate to ephaptic transmission; they last less than two minutes but may occur frequently (sometimes up to 20 to 30 times a day) for a two- to six-week period. They are exquisitely sensitive to carbamazepine, and a small recent study has suggested that gabapentin may be a useful alternative. Bromocriptine also has been mentioned in case reports.

Epilepsy occurs in about 5 percent of people with MS, and although this may be coincidental in some cases, there is evidence to suggest that it relates to either cortical or subcortical lesions or very large plaques that behave like space-occupying lesions and usually occur in advanced disease. Treatment should be with anticonvulsants, although their use need not always be prolonged, particularly if there is only a short cluster of attacks in association with an acute inflammatory lesion that subsequently resolves.

## Cognitive Symptoms

Cognitive deficits occur in up to 60 percent of people with MS and affect attention, conceptual reasoning, executive function, visuospatial perception, and recent memory, with relative sparing of language and intellectual function. They have a major impact on all aspects of functioning, particularly employment, and, not surprisingly, limit the benefits of rehabilitation. Assessment and identification of particular deficits are fundamental to developing strategies to overcome or compensate for the deficits. A cognitive rehabilitation program in which communication skills training was a combination of cognitive rehabilitation and cognitive-behavioral psychotherapy has been described but not yet evaluated. There is little evidence available on the treatment of specific cognitive deficits. The effects of cognitive training and psychotherapy have been evaluated in a small randomized study of 40 patients, but no clear benefit could be determined apart from an apparent improvement in mood in the treatment arm. A computer-based retraining program has been reported to have some short-term benefit (nine weeks) in specific attention deficits in a study of 22 patients. Benefits also were seen in relevant activities of daily living over this period. The only medication to be studied in this regard is 4-aminopyridine, but no significant benefit was seen in a small randomized, double-blind, placebo-controlled, cross-over study of 20 patients.

*In the view of the Committee, these are particularly important symptoms and it is encouraging to see that they are now more widely recognized as such. More active approaches to management are urgently needed.*

## Other Symptoms

### VISUAL DYSFUNCTION

Although optic neuritis, the most common visual symptom, usually is transient and associated with good recovery, some patients have persisting and occasionally progressive deficits and may benefit from referral to a low vision clinic. Involuntary eye movement disorders, such as nystagmus and oscillopsia, also cause distressing visual disturbance. These symptoms may be helped by the use of prisms, and there is anecdotal evidence to suggest the use of a number of medications including baclofen, gabapentin, and isoniazid. A small study has evaluated the role of the glutamate agonist memantine in pendular nystagmus, and all 11 patients treated with this agent showed a positive response.

### VERTIGO

Dizziness or vertigo may occur as part of a brain stem relapse and may be accompanied by nystagmus and ataxia, resulting in a profound reduction in mobility and safety. Prochlorperazine may be helpful in acute vertigo, while physiotherapy, including Cawthorne-Cooksey exercises, together with cinnarazine, may be helpful when symptoms are chronic.

### SWALLOWING, SPEECH, AND RESPIRATORY DYSFUNCTION

Dysphagia is not uncommon in MS, and suggestive symptoms have been reported in up to 43 percent of the MS population. These symptoms included coughing when eating, choking, anxiety about swallowing, and change in swallowing function. Such symptoms are often overlooked until the patient has a severe choking episode. Mild dysphagia usually is easily managed with assessment and advice from a speech therapist. There is a risk of aspiration pneumonia in more severe cases, and investigation may include videofluoroscopy. Percutaneous gastrostomy may be required if swallowing is unsafe or intake is inadequate.

Speech disturbance in MS usually is due to dysarthria, although dysphasia does occasionally occur, usually in patients with severe cognitive deficits. Again, assessment and management by a speech therapist is helpful, and a communication aid may be useful in very severe dysarthria.

Respiratory insufficiency may occur in advanced MS but also may complicate acute brain stem episodes. Respiratory muscle weakness, including diaphragmatic weakness, is the most common cause. Respiratory support may be required in an acute event, while in more chronic situations the patient may be taught to incorporate the diaphragm when talking.

## TEMPERATURE SENSITIVITY

Many patients report a worsening of symptoms associated with an increase in temperature or exercise, particularly in relation to visual function (Uthoff's phenomenon). Practical advice about air-conditioning systems may be helpful, and the use of a cooling suit might be considered if the symptoms are very severe. The drug 4-aminopyridine has been reported to be particularly beneficial in patients with temperature sensitivity.

## PSYCHIATRIC AND PSYCHOLOGICAL DYSFUNCTION

Psychiatric morbidity is increased in MS, with over 50 percent of patients being symptomatic at some stage. Irritability, poor concentration, depressed mood, and anxiety are the most common symptoms. The depressive symptoms often are not severe, and only a minority of patients require medication. The treatment of depression is similar to that for people who do not have MS, and there are few randomized controlled trials of antidepressants in MS. A study of desipramine showed moderate efficacy, but the dose was limited by anticholinergic side effects.

Psychological disturbances are not uncommon in MS, and many patients have difficulty coping from the time of initial diagnosis, which may be compounded by the subsequent development of disability. Different methods for treating psychological difficulties have been described, but few have been evaluated. The role of psychotherapy in MS has been described, and the role of group psychotherapy has been evaluated in a small group of patients with MS. Some benefit was seen in relation to "locus of control," but no effect was seen in anxiety or self-esteem.

*In the view of the Committee, these symptoms need to be actively managed, although this may not involve drug treatment.*

# Neurologic Rehabilitation

The preceding section underlines the wide range of symptoms that may occur in MS, together with the fact that it is usual for many symptoms to coexist and interact. Therefore, any management strategy must take into account how these factors produce a complex pattern of disability, together with the possibility that treating one symptom may worsen another. It also is apparent that comprehensive management will invariably require input from a number of different treatment modalities, including the provision of information, patient education, therapy from a range of disciplines, and drug therapy. Finally, the variable and fluctuating nature of MS means that the needs of the individual patient will change over time, often quite abruptly, and that these needs will tend to increase over time.

The philosophy of rehabilitation, which emphasizes patient education and self-management, is ideally suited to meet the needs of such a complex and progressive disorder as MS. Rehabilitation aims to improve independence and quality of life by minimizing disability and handicap. It has been defined by the World Health Organization as "an active process by which those disabled by injury or disease achieve a full recovery or if a full recovery is not possible realize their optimal physical, mental and social potential and are integrated into their most appropriate environment."

The essential components of successful rehabilitation include:

- Expert multidisciplinary assessment
- Goal-orientated programs
- Evaluation of impact on patient and goal achievement.

## Evaluating Outcome

This component is the most challenging but also the most important if there is to be ongoing improvement in the process and impact of rehabilitation. Evaluating the effect on the patient requires the use of outcome measures that are scientifically sound (reliable, valid, and responsive) and clinically useful (short, simple, etc.). They also must be appropriate to the sample under study and the intervention being evaluated. In the case of neurorehabilitation, the effects are not expected at the levels of pathology and impairment but rather in disability and handicap (or activity and participation as the recently published *International Classification of Impairments, Disabilities, and Handicaps 2* have now suggested) and in the broader, more patient-oriented areas of quality of life, coping skills, and self-efficacy. The standard outcome measure in therapeutic trials in MS, Kurtzke's EDSS is inappropriate for evaluating rehabilitation not only because of its scientific limitations (particularly poor responsiveness) but also because it does not measure many of the relevant areas. Consequently, a number of generic measures of disability (Barthel Index [BI], Functional Independence Measure [FIM], Functional Independence Measure/Functional Assessment Measure [FIM/FAM]), handicap (London Handicap Scale [LHS]), and quality of life (The Short Form 36 Health Survey Questionnaire [SF-36]) have been used in MS rehabilitation (Table 4-2).

More recently, a number of MS-specific measures have been developed that are currently undergoing evaluation and address disability (UK Disability Scale), quality of life (Quality of Life Inventory [LaRocca], Functional Assessment of MS [FAMS], MS QOL 54, The Leeds QOL Scale, and the MS Disease Impact Scale (MSIS).

The evaluation of the rehabilitation process, including goal achievement, may be carried out using integrated care pathways (ICPs). An ICP is an excellent audit tool that documents when goals are not achieved on time but more usefully indicates why this has occurred, such as the underestimation of cognitive dysfunction or the impact of fatigue.

## Evaluating Neurorehabilitation

The difficulties of evaluating any intervention within the context of a randomized, double-blind, placebo-controlled trial in a variable and unpredictable condition such as MS were outlined in Chapter 1. Evaluating as broad an area as neurorehabilitation, which at the same time has to meet the specific needs of an individual patient, poses additional problems in trial design. Chief among these are a lack of detailed description (e.g., number of disciplines involved, techniques employed, etc.) and inadequate standardization of input, including its duration and location (inpatient, outpatient, or community-based). There also is a reluctance among therapists to use a control group, and limited resources often prohibit the use of independent assessors, which is particularly important when blinding is so difficult and perhaps even impossible. Finally, there is no consensus as to the most appropriate outcome measures, and until recently there has been inconsistent use of limited and often inappropriate tools.

Despite these obstacles, it is possible to attempt some degree of evaluation, as has been demonstrated by a number of recent studies, although many more are required. To assess the data these studies have produced, it is useful to consider four distinct levels, moving from the broadest concept of (1) service delivery, to (2) packages of comprehensive rehabilitation, (3) individual components of that package, and, finally, the most specific (4) the intrinsic components of the rehabilitation process (e.g., assessment, goal setting, and so forth—the so-called "black box" of rehabilitation. The majority of studies have focused on comprehensive packages of rehabilitation (predominantly inpatient), but some studies have addressed individual components including physiotherapy and aerobic exercise, and recent studies have compared different forms of delivery of care. There are no published studies on the intrinsic components of rehabilitation as they apply to MS.

## Evaluating Comprehensive Packages of Rehabilitation

The two key questions that need to be answered are:

- Is comprehensive rehabilitation effective in reducing disability, handicap, and quality of life?
- If so, do these benefits carry over in the medium to long term?

The majority of studies have evaluated inpatient rehabilitation, which may be more accessible for study design. Of the eight studies listed in Table 4-3, the earlier four studies are single group design, although all suggest potential benefit from rehabilitation in the area of disability. Two other studies compared inpatient rehabilitation with acute hospital care in a retrospective design and outpatient therapy, respectively. The former suggested there was no difference between the two approaches, while the latter found a marginal benefit from inpatient rehabilitation. The study by Freeman and coworkers was a randomized, wait-list controlled study of 66 patients with progressive MS. Patients were stratified on entry according to EDSS score, and the treatment group received a short period of inpatient rehabilitation (mean, 20 days). Measures of disability, the Functional Independence Measure (FIM), and handicap, the London Handicap Scale (LHS), were applied on entry into the study and six weeks later. The two groups were well matched in relation to age, sex, disease pattern, and duration, and the treated group showed a significant benefit in both disability ($p < 0.001$) and handicap ($p < 0.01$) when compared with the control group. No change in the EDSS score was seen in either group.

A more recent randomized, single-blind trial compared a three-week inpatient rehabilitation program with a home exercise program in 50 less disabled patients who were still ambulatory. Patients were evaluated with the EDSS, FIM, and SF-36, a quality-of-life measure, at baseline, 3, 6, 9,

**Table 4-3** Summary of Outcome Studies of Comprehensive Rehabilitation in People with MS

| Study | Study Design | Sample (n) | Main Outcomes/ Instruments | Time of Assessments | Results |
|---|---|---|---|---|---|
| **Inpatient Rehabilitation** | | | | | |
| Feigenson et al. | Prospective, single group, pre- and post-study design | 20 | Impairment, disability and handicap: MS functional profile (a modified version of BUSTOP) Costs of intervention | Admission and discharge costs were also measured at 12 months (by telephone interview) | Significant benefit in disability and handicap, no change in impairment |
| Greenspan et al. | Retrospective, single group, pre- and post-study design | 28 | Disability: CRDS | Admission, discharge, and 30-month review (by telephone if necessary) | Benefits across a range of disabilities, which were maintained at 3 months |
| Reding et al. | Retrospective study, using case-matched analysis | 20 pairs | Disability: ISS Hospital readmission rate Cost of intervention The need for home assistance | Review at 16 months (by telephone) | No difference between groups |
| Carey et al. | Retrospective multicenter study assessing a range of condition. Single group, pre- and poststudy design | 6194, of whom 196 had MS | Disability: LORS-II | Admission and discharge | Improvements in ADL and mobility |

*continued on next page*

Table 4-3  Summary of Outcome Studies of Comprehensive Rehabilitation in People with MS (continued)

| Study | Study Design | Sample (n) | Main Outcomes/Instruments | Time of Assessments | Results |
|---|---|---|---|---|---|
| **Inpatient Rehabilitation** | | | | | |
| Francabandera et al. | Prospective, stratified, randomized study | 84 | Disability: ISS; Need for home assistance (hours) | Admission and at 3-month intervals for 2 years (3-month results reported in this publication) | Preliminary results suggest marginal benefit in inpatient group |
| Kidd et al. | Prospective, single group, pre- and poststudy design | 79 | Impairment: DSS; Disability: Barthel Index; Handicap: ESS | Admission and discharge | Statistically significant improvement in disability and handicap |
| Freeman et al. | Prospective, single group, longitudinal study design | 50 (all in the prog. stage) | Impairment: FS and EDSS; Disability: FIM; Handicap: LHS; Quality of life: SF-36; Emotional well-being: GHQ-28 | Admission and discharge and at 3-month intervals for 1 year | Benefits in disability, handicap, QoL, and emotional well-being persist for 6–9 months |
| Solari et al. | Randomized single group study comparing inpatient and home exercise program | 50 (ambulatory) | Impairment: EDSS; Disability: FIM; Quality of life: SF-36 | Baseline, 3, 9, and 15 weeks | Benefits in disability and some aspects of QoL |

*continued on next page*

Table 4-3 Summary of Outcome Studies of Comprehensive Rehabilitation in People with MS (continued)

| Study | Study Design | Sample (n) | Main Outcomes/ Instruments | Time of Assessments | Results |
|---|---|---|---|---|---|
| **Carry over** | | | | | |
| Aisen et al. | Retrospective, single group, pre- and poststudy design | 37 | Impairment: FS and EDSS<br>Disability: FIM | Admission, discharge, and telephone follow-up (between 6 and 36 months post discharge) | Significant improvement in both FIM and EDSS |
| Kidd, Thompson | Prospective, single group, pre- and poststudy design | 47 | Impairment: EDSS<br>Disability: FIM<br>Handicap: ESS | Admission, discharge, and 3-month follow-up | Gains in disability maintained at 3 months handicap improved over study period |
| Freeman et al. | Stratified, randomized, wait list controlled study design | 66 (all in the prog. stage) | Impairment: FS and EDSS<br>Disability: FIM<br>Handicap: LHS | Baseline and 6 weeks | Significant benefit in disability and handicap |
| **Outpatient Rehabilitation** | | | | | |
| Di Fabio et al. | Nonequivalent pre-test, post-test control group design | 45 with prog MS | MS-related symptom RIC-FAS<br>Fatigue frequency | At entry and at one year | 33 patients completed one year<br>Significant benefit seen in MS-related symptoms, inc. fatigue |

BUSTOP: Burke Stroke Time-oriented Profile; CRDS: Computerized Rehabilitation and Data System; DSS: Disability Status Scale; EDSS: Expanded Disability Status Scale; ESS: Environmental Status Scale; FIM: Functional Independence Measure; LORS-II: Revised Level of Rehabilitation Scale; FS: Functional Systems; ISS: Incapacity Status Scale; LHS: London Handicap Scale; SF-36: Short Form 36 Health Survey Questionnaire; GHQ-28: 28-item General Health Questionnaire; RIC-FAS: Rehabilitation Institute of Chicago, Functional Assessment Scale.

and 15 weeks. Significant benefit in disability and some aspects of quality of life (mental not physical) was seen at the end of the three-week period in the rehabilitation group compared with those doing a home exercise program. This beneficial difference between groups was seen again at 9 weeks but had disappeared by 15 weeks.

Few researchers have attempted to evaluate outpatient-based rehabilitation in MS, but a study by Di Fabio and colleagues randomly assigned 46 patients with progressive MS to an active treatment group (20 patients receiving 5 hours of outpatient therapy a week for one year) and to a wait-list control group. The range of outcomes used included an MS-related symptoms checklist composite score, a measure of fatigue frequency, and items from the Rehabilitation Institute of Chicago's Functional Assessment Scale. A significant reduction in the frequency of MS symptoms and fatigue was seen.

**Conclusion:** *Although it is difficult to combine the results of all of these studies and there are major methodological differences between them, with few, if any, reaching an adequate scientific level, they all suggest that organized patient-centered multidisciplinary rehabilitation is of benefit in MS management. The degree of benefit and the extent of carryover have yet to be determined.*

## Do Benefits of Rehabilitation Carry Over in Medium Term?

Three studies have attempted to address this question over the last three years with varying degrees of success and all of which were restricted to the evaluation of a single group. The first was a retrospective study based on reviewing inpatient records and making subsequent phone contact with 37 patients 6 to 36 months later. It suggested that gains on the EDSS and FIM documented on discharge were maintained at follow-up. The second study was a prospective evaluation of 47 patients seen 3 months post discharge and included a measure of handicap (Environmental Status Scale) along with the EDSS and FIM. No change was seen in the EDSS during or following rehabilitation; gains in the FIM were maintained, while the level of handicap actually improved over the three-month follow-up period.

The most recent study involved the prospective longitudinal evaluation of 50 of the patients with progressive MS involved in the randomized control trial described earlier. This study used a wider range of outcome measures; in addition to the EDSS and FIM, there were measures of handicap (LHS), quality of life (SF-36), and emotional well-being (General Health Questionnaire GHQ). Patients were evaluated for 12 months at 3-month intervals following discharge, and 12-month data were collected on 48 of the 50 patients (92%). As might be expected, there was great variation between individual patients as well as considerable differences between the outcome measures. Summary measures were used to calculate the time taken to return to baseline. The EDSS deteriorated from a median of 6.8 on discharge to 8.0 at 12-month follow-up. Despite this, the gains in disability were maintained for 6 months before slowly declining. As in the previous study, handicap improved further following discharge, but the benefit lessened after 6 months. Quality of life and emotional well-being improved considerably during the rehabilitation period, and this improvement was maintained for 10 and 7 months, respectively, before beginning to return to the baseline. A further finding of this study was that those who made the most gains during the rehabilitation period tended to maintain those gains for a longer time.

**Conclusion:** *Despite their methodological limitations, these studies provide some evidence to suggest that the gains derived from rehabilitation are maintained in the short term, at least in part, in this progressive condition. They emphasize the need for a range of outcome measures to be used and stress the importance a continuity of care following discharge into the community.*

## Evaluating Components of the Rehabilitation Package

Few studies have looked at therapy intervention in the management of MS, and the only specific modality examined has been physiotherapy. A randomized control trial of inpatient physiotherapy (6.5 hours over 2 weeks) was carried out on 45 patients. Outcome measures included the Rivermead Mobility Index, the Barthel ADL Index, and a visual analogue scale (VAS) of "mobility-related distress"; the only measure to demonstrate a significant benefit in the treated group was the VAS. However, the same authors recently demonstrated a significant benefit from outpatient or domiciliary physiotherapy. A second study went a step further and attempted to compare two forms of physiotherapy. This pilot study involved 23 patients, 20 of whom completed the study. Ten patients received what was described as an impairment-based "facilitation approach" (e.g., Bobath), while the other group had a more disability-based task-orientated approach (e.g., Carr and Shepherd). Patients received a minimum of 15 sessions over 5 to 7 weeks. The outcome measures were mobility-based and included the 10-meter timed walk and the Rivermead Mobility Index. Not surprisingly, no difference was seen between the two small groups, but both improved from baseline (p < 0.05). A recent randomized, controlled, cross-over study evaluated hospital and home-based physiotherapy in 40 MS patients with mobility problems. A very wide range of outcome measures was used, but physiotherapy resulted in signifcant benefit, irrespective of location, on the Rivermead Mobility Index, which was supported by other measures of mobility, gait, and balance. There was no difference between treatment at home (the patients's preference) or in the hospital, although the latter was less expensive.

The impact of aerobic exercise was evaluated in 46 patients with relatively mild MS. Twenty-one patients were randomly assigned to a 15-week exercise program, while 25 patients had no exercise during that period. There was a wide range of outcome measures, including aerobic capacity, isometric strength, a quality-of-life measure, the Sickness Impact Profile (SIP), the Fatigue Severity Scales (FSS), and the EDSS. Significant changes from baseline were seen in the exercise group over the 15 weeks in the physiologic measures and the physical component of the SIP. There was little sustained change in the psychosocial domain of the SIP and none in the EDSS or FSS.

**Conclusion:** *There is a paucity of evidence to support the role of therapy in MS, but recent studies have confirmed that such studies are now feasible and urgently need to be carried out.*

## Evaluating Service Delivery

Evaluating service delivery may be considered the most important and relevant issue in the management of MS because it incorporates acute hospital and neurorehabilitation services together with community-based activities and, in essence, has to bring together medical and social services in a way that meets the complex and ever-changing needs of the person with MS. The key components of such a service include:

- Support at diagnostic phase
- High level of expertise
- Comprehensive, flexible
- Accessible, coordinated

■ Linked to neuroscience center

Subsequently, many of these have been incorporated into standards of care that identify the key issues and standards applicable to them at each of four stages of the condition: diagnostic, minimal impairment, moderate disability, and severe disability. Ideally, most services should be community-based with supporting expertise from the acute hospital or rehabilitation center at times of particular need (e.g., at diagnosis or at the time of a severe relapse) or complexity (when multiple symptoms interact and intensive inpatient rehabilitation is required). The optimum method of service delivery has not yet been defined, and little work has been done comparing existing services. A recently completed, although not yet published, study carried out in Rome compared two forms of service delivery in a randomized controlled trial of 201 patients with MS. One group (133 patients) received what was described as "hospital" home care, in which patients remained in the community but had immediate access to the hospital-based multidisciplinary team as and when required, while the other group (68 patients) received routine care. The range of outcomes, which included EDSS, FIM, SF-36, and measures of anxiety and mood, were carried out at baseline and at 12 months. No difference was seen in the level of disability between the two groups, but the more intensively treated patients had significantly less depression and improved quality of life. Another study comparing the benefits of multidisciplinary MS clinics, general neurology outpatients, and community-based general practice in 150 patients (50 in each group) has just commenced in the United Kingdom. Patients will be evaluated at baseline and at 3-month intervals for 1 year with a range of outcome measures from impairment to self-efficacy.

**Conclusion:** *Although there is good empirical evidence to support coordinated expert service delivery, there is little evidence currently available to support this concept in the management of MS, and further studies are required.*

# References

## General Reviews

■ Thompson AJ. Symptomatic treatment in multiple sclerosis. *Curr Opin Neurol* 1998; 11:305–309.

- Kesselring J, Thompson AJ. Spasticity, ataxia and fatigue in multiple sclerosis. In: Miller DH (ed). *Bailliére's Clinical Neurology. International Practice and Research: Multiple Sclerosis*. London: Bailliere Tindall, 1997.
- Schapiro RT, Baumhefner RW, Tourtellotte WW. Multiple sclerosis: A clinical viewpoint to management. In: Raine CS, McFarland HF, Tourtellotte WW. *Multiple Sclerosis: Clinical and Pathogenetic Base*. London: Chapman and Hall, 1997.

## Spasticity

- Sheean G. Pathophysiology of spasticity. In: Sheean G (ed.). *Spasticity Rehabilitation*. Edinburgh: Churchill Communications Europe Ltd., 1998:17–38.
- Barnes MP. Local treatment of spasticity. In: *Baillière's Clinical Neurology*. Vol. 2. London: Baillière Tindall 1993:55–71.
- Thompson AJ. Spasticity rehabilitation: A rational approach to clinical management. In: Sheean G (ed.). *Spasticity Rehabilitation*. Edinburgh: Churchill Communications Europe Ltd., 1998:51–56.
- Hattab JR. Review of European clinical trials with baclofen. In: Feldman RG, Young RR, Koella WP (eds.). *Spasticity: Disordered Motor Control*. Chicago: Year Book; 1980:71–85.
- Wagstaff AJ, Bryson HM. Tizanidine: A review of its pharmacology, clinical efficacy and tolerability in the management of spasticity associated with cerebral and spinal disorders. *Drugs* 1997; 53(3):435–452.
- Bakheit AMO. Management of muscle spasticity. *Crit Rev Phys Med Rehab* 1996; 8(3):235–252.
- Penn RD, Savoy SM, Corcos D, et al. Intrathecal baclofen for severe spinal spasticity. *N Engl J Med* 1989; 320:1517–1521.
- Ochs G, Struppler A, Meyerson BA, et al. Intrathecal baclofen for long-term treatment of spasticity: A multi-centre study. *J Neurol Neurosurg Psychiatry* 1989; 52:933–939.
- Hymen N, Barnes B, Bhakta B, et al. Botulinum toxin treatment of hip adductor spasticity in multiple sclerosis: A prospective, randomised, double blind, placebo controlled dose ranging study. *J Neurol Neurosurg Psychiatry* 2000; 68:707–712.

## Ataxia

- Alusi SH, Glickman S, Aziz TZ, Bain PG. Tremor in multiple sclerosis. *J Neurol Neurosurg Psychiatry* 1999; 66:131–134. Editorial.
- Hallett M, Lindsey JW, Adelstein BD, Riley PO. Controlled trial of isoniazid therapy for severe postural cerebellar tremor in multiple sclerosis. *Neurology* 1985; 35(9):1374–1377.
- Koller WC. Pharmacologic trials in the treatment of cerebellar tremor. *Arch Neurol* 1984; 41:280–281.
- Rice GPA, Lescaux J, Ebers G. Ondansetron versus placebo for disabling cerebellar tremor: Final report of a randomized clinical trial. *Ann Neurol* 1999; 46:493.

- Montgomery EB, Baker KB, Kinkel RP, Barnett G. Chronic thalamic stimulation for the tremor of multiple sclerosis. *Neurology* 1999; 53:625–628.
- Schuurman PR, Andries Bosch D, Bossuyt PMM, et al. A comparison of continuous thalamic stimulation and thalamotomy for suppression of severe tremor. *N Engl J Med* 2000; 342:461–468.

## Fatigue

- Krupp LB. Mechanisms, measurement, and management of fatigue in multiple sclerosis. In: Thompson AJ, Polman C, Hohlfeld R (eds.). *Multiple Sclerosis: Clinical Challenges and Controversies*. London: Martin Dunitz, 1997:283–294.
- Krupp LB, Coyle PK, Doscher C, et al. Fatigue therapy in multiple sclerosis: Results of a double-blind, randomized, parallel trial of amantadine, pemoline, and placebo. *Neurology* 1995; 45(11):1956–1961.
- van Diemen HA, Polman CH, van Dongen TM, et al. The effect of 4-aminopyridine on clinical signs in multiple sclerosis: A randomized, placebo-controlled, double-blind, cross-over study. *Ann Neurol* 1992; 32(2):123–130.
- Multiple Sclerosis Council for Clinical Practice Guidelines. Fatigue and Multiple Sclerosis. Washington, DC: Paralyzed Veterans of America, 1998.

## Bladder Dysfunction

- MS Council for Clinical Practice Guidelines. Urinary Dysfunction and Multiple Sclerosis. Evidence-Based Management Strategies for Urinary Dysfunction in Multiple Sclerosis. Washington, DC: Paralyzed Veterans of America, 1998.
- Betts CD, D'Mellow MT, Fowler CJ. Urinary symptoms and the neurological features of bladder dysfunction in multiple sclerosis. *J Neurol Neurosurg Psychiatry* 1993; 56(3):245–250.
- Fowler CJ. Investigation of the neurogenic bladder. *J Neurol Neurosurg Psychiatry* 1996; 60:6–13.
- Valiquette G, Herbert J, Maede D. Desmopressin in the management of nocturia in patients with multiple sclerosis. A double-blind, crossover trial. *Arch Neurol* 1996; 53:1270–1275.
- Vahtera T, Haaranen M, Viramo-Koskela AL, Ruutiainen J. Pelvic floor rehabilitation is effective in patients with multiple sclerosis. *Clin Rehabil* 1997; 11:211–219.

## Bowel Dysfunction

- Hinds JP, Eidelman BH, Wald A. Prevalence of bowel dysfunction in MS. *Gastroenterology* 1990; 98:1538–1542.
- Fowler CJ, Henry MM. Gastrointestinal dysfunction in MS. *Semin Neurol* 1996; 16:277–279.

## Sexual Dysfunction

- Zorzon M, Zivadinov R, Bosco A, et al. Sexual dysfunction in multiple sclerosis: A case-control study. 1. Frequency and comparison of groups. *Multiple Sclerosis* 1999; 5:418–427.
- Betts CD, Jones SJ, Fowler CG, Fowler CJ. Erectile dysfunction in multiple sclerosis. Associated neurological and neurophysiological deficits, and treatment of the condition. *Brain* 1994; 117:1303–1310.

## Pain

- Archibald CJ, McGrath, PJ, Ritvo PG, et al. Pain prevalence, severity and impact in a clinic sample of multiple sclerosis patients. *Pain* 1994; 58:89–93.
- Reder AT, Arnason BGW. Trigeminal neuralgia in multiple sclerosis relieved by a prostaglandin E analogue. *Neurology* 1995; 45:1097–1100.
- Khan OA. Gabapentin relieves trigeminal neuralgia in multiple sclerosis patients. *Neurology* 1998; 51:611–614.
- Broggi G, Ferroli P, Franzini A, Servello D, Dones I. Microvascular decompression for trigeminal neuralgia: Comments on a series of 250 cases, including 10 patients with multiple sclerosis. *J Neurol Neurosurg Psychiatry* 2000; 68:59–64.

## Cognitive Dysfunction

- Rao SM, Leo GJ, Ellington L, et al. Cognitive dysfunction in multiple sclerosis. II. Impact on employment and social functioning. *Neurology* 1991; 41:692–696.
- Jonnsson A, Korfitzen EM, Heltberg A, Ravnborg MH, Byskov-Ottosen, E. Effects of neuropsychological treatment in patients with multiple sclerosis. *Acta Neurol Scand* 1993; 88:394–400.
- Plohmann AM, Kappos L, Ammann W, et al. Computer assisted retraining of attentional impairments in patients with multiple sclerosis. *J Neurol Neurosurg Psychiatry* 1998; 64:455–462.

## Visual, Swallowing, and Respiratory Dysfunction

- Starck M, Albrecht H, Pollmann W, Straube A, Dieterich M. Drug therapy for acquired pendular nystagmus in multiple sclerosis. *J Neurol* 1997; 244:9–16.
- Abraham S, Scheinberg LC, Smith CR, LaRocca NG. Neurologic impairment and disability status in outpatients with multiple sclerosis reporting dysphagia symptomatology. *J Neuro Rehab* 1997; 11(1):7–13.
- Howard RS, Wiles CM, Hirsch NP, et al. Respiratory involvement in multiple sclerosis. *Brain* 1992; 115:479–494.

## Psychiatric and Psychological Dysfunction

- Ron MA, Logsdail SJ. Psychiatric morbidity in multiple sclerosis: A clinical and MRI study. *Psychol Med* 1989; 19:887–895.

## Neurorehabilitation

- Thompson AJ, Hobart JC. Multiple sclerosis: Assessment of disability and disability scales. *J Neurol* 1998; 245(4):189–196.
- Jonsson A, Dock J, Ravnborg MH. Quality of life as a measure of rehabilitation outcome in patients with multiple sclerosis. *Acta Neurol Scand* 1996; 93:229–235.
- Sharrack B, Hughes RAC, Soudain S, Dunn G. The psychometric properties of clinical rating scales used in multiple sclerosis. *Brain* 1999; 122:141–160.
- Fischer JS, LaRocca NG, Miller DM, et al. Recent developments in the assessment of quality of life in multiple sclerosis (MS). *Multiple Sclerosis* 1999; 5:251–260.
- Cella DF, Dineen K, Arnason B, et al. Validation of the functional assessment of multiple sclerosis quality of life instrument. *Neurology* 1996; 47(1): 129–139.
- Vickrey BG, Hays RD, Harooni R, Myers LW, Ellison GW. A health-related quality of life measure for multiple sclerosis. *Qual Life Res* 1995; 4(3): 187–206.
- Rossiter DA, Edmondson A, Al-Shahi R, Thompson AJ. Integrated care pathways in multiple sclerosis: Completing the audit cycle. *Multiple Sclerosis* 1998; 4:85–89.
- Jonsson A, Ravnborg MH. Rehabilitation in multiple sclerosis. *Phys Rehab Med* 1998; 10(1):75–100.
- Freeman JA, Langdon DW, Hobart JC, Thompson AJ. The impact of inpatient rehabilitation on progressive multiple sclerosis. *Ann Neurol* 1997; 42(2):236–244.
- Solari A, Filippini G, Gasco P, et al. Physical rehabilitation has a positive effect on disability in multiple sclerosis patients. *Neurology* 1999; 52(1): 57–62.
- Di Fabio RP, Soderberg J, Choi T, Hansen CR, Schapiro RT. Extended outpatient rehabilitation: Its influence on symptom frequency, fatigue and functional status for persons with progressive multiple sclerosis. *Arch Phys Med Rehabil* 1998; 79(2):141–146.
- Aisen ML, Sevilla D, Fox N. Inpatient rehabilitation for multiple sclerosis. *J Neuro Rehab* 1996; 10:43–46.
- Freeman JA, Langdon DW, Hobart JC, Thompson AJ. Inpatient rehabilitation in multiple sclerosis: Do the benefits carry over into the community? *Neurology* 1999; 52:50–56.
- Petajan JH, Gappmaier E, White AT, et al. Impact of aerobic training on fitness and quality of life in multiple sclerosis. *Ann Neurol* 1996; 39(4):432–441.
- Hatch J, Johnson J, Thompson AJ. Standards of health care for people with MS. *MS Management* 1999; 5:16–25.
- Pozzilli C, Pisani A, Palmisano L, Battaglia MA, Fieschi C, and the Roman Home Care Multiple Sclerosis Group. Service location in multiple sclerosis: Home or hospital. In: Fredrikson S, Link H (eds.). *Advances in Multiple*

*Sclerosis: Clinical Research and Therapy.* London: Martin Dunitz. 1999: 173–180.

- Wiles CM, Newcombe RG, Fuller KJ, et al. A controlled, randomised, crossover trial of the effects of physiotherapy on mobility on chronic multiple sclerosis. *J Neurol Neurosurg Psychiatry* 2001; 70:174–179.

# CHAPTER 5

# Alternative Therapies
# Used by People with MS

The previous sections in this book mostly record conventional therapies used by physicians after they have been studied and tested using scientific methods and clinical trials. Therapies such as the interferons or tizanidine are subject to rigorous study and clinical trials before they are approved for treatment of MS, and even then only for use in defined circumstances.

*Randomized clinical trials* (RCT) are used to evaluate the effect of a potential treatment, and careful statistical evaluation determines the benefits and the risks. Although the RCT is the "gold standard" for assessing therapy in MS and other diseases, there are many approaches and agents that are not often subjected to such regulation and clinical trials. Such approaches include herbal medicine, health food supplements, and spiritual healing methods. It is not that such approaches are necessarily of no value, but they are mostly unproven. They may produce comfort or ease of symptoms, or they may evoke the *placebo response*, in which the patient feels better because a therapy is being used rather than from the therapy itself.

The dividing line between *conventional medicine* provided by physicians and hospitals and *alternative* or *complementary medicine* is not always clear-cut, but in this section we explain the approaches of both systems and some of the types of alternative and complementary medical approaches commonly used by people with MS.

The use of alternative medicines is not new. In earlier centuries physicians made wide use of herbs, plants, massage, and hydrotherapy, as well as astrology, in attempts to heal and comfort patients, very much like the alternative therapies of today. As more was learned about the causes and mechanisms of disease, newer approaches were used, and those therapies that could not be shown to help were put aside. The scientific age brought with it a way of testing a hypothesis and looking at evidence in an objective and critical way. There also was an acceptance that constant critique and inquiry would cause knowledge and approaches to continually change. Thus everything is subject to question, and the hope would be that change would bring about new and better approaches to treatment.

Medicine is based in science and has a basis in critical analysis and constant change, replacing old or unfounded ideas and concepts with new ones based on new knowledge and research. In most alternative therapies, there is a basis in *belief*, a reluctance to challenge the belief, and resistance to change. This is understandable as a practitioner of a single approach, such as therapeutic touch, would be reluctant to challenge or objectively examine whether therapeutic touch was effective or greater than the placebo effect because it would call into question the entire belief.

## Definition of Alternative or Complementary Medicine

Many terms have been applied to a wide variety of approaches that have their origins in different theories, philosophies, and religions. None is satisfactory, but commonly used terms are *alternative, complementary, empirical, unconventional, integrative,* and *holistic,* or terms that are pejorative, such as *fringe, nonscientific, unproven,* or *"quack"* remedies.

*Alternative* implies choosing a different approach to health and illness than conventional and scientific medicine; in other words, a parallel but different system. Thus one might chose, for example, Christian Science or homeopathy as a way of understanding and treating illness, rejecting much or all of conventional medicine.

*Complementary* implies a form of therapy that is used *along with* conventional medicine. This could be vitamin and health food supplements, meditation, magnetism, or astrology used along with conventional medicine. The person may accept conventional medicine but add other approaches and medicines that are not part of it.

The National Institutes of Health (NIH) in the United States has grouped these two together into complementary and alternative medicine

(CAM). This groups many different approaches, some of which may be incompatible with the others. They are grouped because they are not "mainstream medicine" or are not traditionally taught in medical schools.

This separation into alternative or complementary forms is artificial for many reasons. Some approaches used to be mainstream medicine (herbs and purging were used for many centuries by physicians), and now many medical schools provide courses to make medical students aware of alternative medicine. Additionally, because it is the nature of medicine to examine, assess, and constantly change, therapies that were mainstream in the past may be discarded when found to be of little benefit, whereas others, including alternative approaches, will be accepted if studies show conclusively that they are safe and beneficial.

In this section we refer to these therapies as alternative medicine.

## The Popularity of Alternative Medicine

In the United States and Canada about one-third of the healthy population will use an alternative therapy or therapists in any year. This appears to be increasing, as is noticeable by the expanding sections of over-the-counter (OTC) medicines in pharmacies, the development of increasing numbers of health food stores and outlets, and advertisements for more and new forms of therapies. The total annual expenditure for alternative medicines in the United States is over $27 billion dollars. Many people are turning to alternative medicines not because they are sick but because they want to stay healthy or because they feel under stress.

The use of alternative medicine is even greater in people with a chronic disease. In many studies of MS, three-fourths of the people use one or more therapies or visit alternative therapists. Although studies have shown that there are certain groups of people with MS who may use alternative medicines more, suffice it to say that it is common by a large number regardless of age, gender, state of health, education, or income. A Danish study suggests that the use of alternative medicines declines as the disease progresses.

Some believe that alternative medicines are more likely to be "natural" and thus freer of side effects, but this is not necessarily true. Again the lines are blurred, as many alternative medicines are manufactured and processed and as "unnatural" as any other drugs, and many conventional medicines produced by the pharmaceutical industry are natural products (probably 25%). Many alternative and natural remedies do have side effects and risks, and people should be aware of these before embarking on any therapy, whether conventional or alternative.

The media promote interest in various therapies by overemphasizing "cures" or "breakthroughs," often illustrated by a case history. Such overemphasized anecdotes are written about both conventional therapies and alternative therapies. Such stories are often premature and the claims exaggerated. A common pattern is a story about a "new treatment for MS" when a potential agent is just about to undergo a clinical trial. The trial is to show whether it is useful and if it should be a treatment. There also are the anecdotal stories about someone who has been very weakened by MS and then is able to get out of the wheelchair when treated with the newest fad therapy. Recovering from an MS attack of severe symptoms and paralysis often happens without treatment, so judgments based on anecdotes are often misguided.

Both conventional medicine and alternative therapies constitute multibillion dollar businesses, but only one is routinely controlled and regulated and required to provide evidence of efficacy as medicine. Qualifications vary from one jurisdiction to another. Some practitioners of therapies require specific education and qualification, and others are therapists because they say they have a treatment form to offer. Acceptance by insurance agencies vary, and this also varies in different jurisdictions. Some alternative therapies are regulated and licensed, but most are not.

## Informing Your Doctor

Most people who use alternative medicines or go to alternative therapists do not inform their physicians of this, sometimes because they think these are not "drugs," or that they are a separate personal activity, or because they believe the doctors will be judgmental and critical. However, there is a lot of evidence that most physicians are not as negative as their patients suspect. Studies of medical students show that many of them are very positive about various forms of alternative medicines and practices, and many will incorporate aspects of it into their practices. Two-thirds of American medical schools provide courses on complementary and alternative medicine for their medical students. A study in Britain showed that more than half the general practitioners provide access to alternative therapies from their practices, and some do them in the practice or have staff or visiting staff perform them. A meta-analysis of all the surveys of doctors showed that doctors generally believe that alternative therapies can be moderately effective and that younger physicians were more positive than older physicians. However, physicians are often cautious about therapies that have not been proven, and the International Code of Medicine Ethics advises a doctor to exercise great caution in using methods of treatment whose value is not recognized by the profession.

The NIH has formed the National Center for Complementary and Alternative Medicine (NCCAM) and has allotted $50 million to support research protocols about CAM. The Association of Canadian Medical Colleges has formed a Special Interest Group on CAM. In Britain there is the Research Council for Complementary Medicine (60 Great Ormond St., London WC1N 3JF, UK). The Tzu Chi Institute for Complementary and Alternative Medicine was opened at the Vancouver General Hospital in Canada in 1996, and the Department of Health in England helps fund the Center for Complementary Medicine at Exeter University. There is a new journal devoted to the studies of alternative medicine, *Scientific Review of Alternative Medicine.*

This chapter describes more than 50 treatments that have been claimed to be of benefit in MS. The rationale for many of them is nonexistent or weak, based on current scientific principles and what we now know about MS. Only a few have undergone a controlled trial.

Some of the methods outlined in this chapter have clearly been the subject of commercial exploitation. Unfortunately, there are many instances in which clinics promote a specific "treatment" that is, in fact, of unproven value. Such clinics thrive on the very natural frustration and desperation of some people with MS and exploit the high likelihood of a placebo response. Anecdotes of dramatic success maintain the reputation of many such clinics.

There is no doubt that an appropriate combination of comforting physical and spiritual activity can do much to stimulate a positive coping attitude in people with MS and contribute to improvement in activities of daily living.

The Medical Management Committee advocates that people with MS respond to claims for a new (or old) treatment for their disease only if (1) they have sought information about what the therapy is and what studies are published to substantiate the claims, (2) they have discussed the therapy with their physician to ensure that it is safe in combination with other therapies the patient is taking, and (3) the cost of treatment does not unnecessarily strain their financial resources.

Table 5-1   Commonly Used Therapies and Therapists

| | |
|---|---|
| Acupressure | Jin Shin Jyutsu |
| Acupuncture | Light Therapy |
| Alexander Technique | Magnetism |
| Applied Kinesiology | Maharishi Ayurveda |
| Aromatherapy | Muscle Therapy |
| Aston Patterning | Naprapathy |
| Ayurvedic Medicine | Naturopathic Medicine |
| Barbara Brennan Healing Science | Neurolinguistic Programming |
| Bioenergetics | Neuromuscular Therapy |
| Biofeedback | Ohashiatsu |
| Bonnie Pruden Myotherapy | Ortho-Bionomy |
| Cervicolordodesis | Osteopathy |
| Chelation | Pilates Method |
| Chi Gong | Polarity Therapy |
| Chinese Oriental Medicine | Pranayama |
| Chiropractic | Qigong |
| Chiropractic Network | Rebirthing |
| Craniocervical Therapy | Reflexology |
| Curanderismo | Regression/Past-Life Therapy |
| Deep Tissue Bodywork | Reiki |
| Do-in | Rolfing |
| Esalen Massage | Rosen Method |
| Feldenkrais Method | Rubenfeld Synergy Method |
| Flower Essences (Bach Flower) | Shiatsu |
| Focusing | Soma Neuromuscular Integration |
| Guided Imagery | Structural Integration |
| Hellerwork | Swedish Massage |
| Herbalism | Tai Chi |
| Holistic Medicine | Therapeutic Touch |
| Holistic Psychotherapy/Counseling | Trager Method |
| Homeopathy | Trigger Point Therapy |
| Hydrotherapy | Western Herbalism |
| Hypnotherapy | Yoga |
| Iridology | Zero Balancing |
| Jin Shin Do Body/Mind Acupressure | |

# Miscellaneous Empirical Treatments

## Injected Materials

### INTRAVENOUS YEASTS (PROPER-MYL)

**Description:** A preparation of cells from three species of yeast; administered intravenously.

**Rationale:** It has been claimed that Proper-myl augments bodily defenses against infections and allergic reactions. It may be expected to act biologically much like typhoid vaccine.

**Evaluation:** As is often true, early reports were encouraging, but later reports showed results no better than known ineffective "treatments" for MS.

**Risks/Costs:** Occasional mild fever.

**Conclusion:** On the basis of published data, Proper-myl appears to be ineffective in the treatment of MS.

> *In the opinion of the Committee, there appears to be no generally accepted scientific basis for use of this therapy. It has never been tested in a properly controlled trial. Risks are undetermined.*

### PANCREATIC EXTRACT (DEPROPANEX)

**Description:** A preparation derived from beef pancreas; given intramuscularly. The exact composition is not known, but it does not contain protein.

**Rationale:** Depropanex was used in MS treatment because it was considered to have both a vasodilating effect and an influence on carbohydrate metabolism.

**Evaluation:** In a small uncontrolled series, most people were considered improved, whereas one patient was unchanged and one patient worsened. Improvement was chiefly in speech, spasticity, and general feeling of well-being, but was not very impressive. Disease progression was not prevented.

**Risks/Costs:** If injected repeatedly, foreign large molecules may induce severe, sometimes life-threatening reactions.

**Conclusion:** On the basis of the limited data, this treatment cannot be considered effective in MS.

*In the opinion of the Committee, this therapy has been adequately tested and shown to be without value. Risks are undetermined.*

### HEART AND PANCREAS EXTRACT (PANCORPHEN)

**Description:** A weak protein solution prepared by digesting beef heart with hog pancreas. It was used as a culture medium for growing bacteria.

**Rationale:** A similar culture medium had been used to grow bacteria in the preparation of a vaccine used to treat MS in 1930 (Purves-Stewart vaccine), which was ineffective.

**Evaluation:** Pancorphen was administered intravenously. Immediate worsening of neurologic symptoms occurred and lasted varying times, from hours to two weeks.

**Risks/Costs:** In addition to worsening of neurologic symptoms, general symptoms of fatigue, shortness of breath, hives, edema, and eczema occurred.

**Conclusion:** Pancorphen appears unacceptable as a treatment for MS because there is no evidence of benefit, and there is evidence of side effects and an adverse effect on MS symptoms..

*In the opinion of the Committee, this therapy should not be used because of reported harmful effects.*

### SNAKE VENOM (PROVEN, VENOGEN, HORVI MS9)

**Description:** PROven is a processed mixture of cobra, krait, and water moccasin venoms for subcutaneous injection. It has been spectrographically analyzed, but its exact composition has not been established. It appears to contain many proteins and some of the numerous enzymatic activities of the original venoms used in the mixture.

**Rationale:** The original idea for using snake venom in MS treatment occurred when a person who worked with snakes was bitten by a krait. Among the neurologic symptoms he suffered were some that suggested stimulation of the nervous system. Subsequently, there were many additional suggestions: that PROven might act as an immune stimulant, might prevent the action of a slow or persistent virus, or might act because of the nerve growth factor that it contains. Claims are also made that PROven reduces inflammation and pain. None of these claims have been investigated scientifically. PROven has also been suggested as a treatment for arthritis and lupus, herpes simplex, herpes zoster, muscular dystrophy, Parkinson's disease, myasthenia gravis, and amyotrophic lateral sclerosis (ALS).

**Evaluation:** Patients initially receive 20 injections and continue the injections at home. The follow-up is chiefly by letters or phone calls from patients who believe they have been helped. There is no attempt to seek patients who have not shown improvement. There have been no reports of objective or quantified examination to document any changes. The U.S. Food and Drug Administration (FDA) has banned the sale of snake venom for the treatment of MS and arthritis until it is tested for safety and effectiveness. PROven continues to be dispensed by several Florida physicians. A similar mixture known as Horvi MS9 (or Horvi Psy 4 or Harviton) is sold in drugstores in Germany. An earlier mixture, Venogen, is no longer on the market.

**Risks/Costs:** Pain and swelling are induced at the injection site. These tend to diminish as the injections are repeated over days to weeks. One severe allergic reaction to PROven has been reported. One young woman receiving PROven injections died of an unusual type of brain hemorrhage.

**Conclusion:** There are no objective controlled studies. The lack of standardized preparation of known composition and proven safety precludes clinical trials at this time. Based on the evidence examined, this treatment is not recommended.

> *In the opinion of the Committee, there appears to be no generally accepted scientific basis for use of this therapy. It has never been tested in a properly controlled trial. Its use carries significant risk.*

### Honey Bee Venom

Although perhaps unrelated in terms of potential mechanism, the benefits of honey bee venom has been the subject of many anecdotal reports from individuals with MS. There are no clinical studies to demonstrate the safety or efficacy of this treatment.

**Description:** Extracts of the bee venom.

**Rationale:** This was an old folk remedy, particularly in New England, first used in treating rheumatic conditions. It was theorized by its advocates that it stimulated the immune system and thus might be useful in MS.

**Evaluation:** There is no evidence that it is an effective treatment for MS. The National MS Society in the United States has funded some laboratory studies to determine whether there is evidence of immune effect in animals, but no patient trials have been considered to be worthwhile.

**Risks/Costs:** There is a risk of severe allergic reaction, as may occur with natural bee stings. There is considerable discomfort if real bees are used and mild discomfort if a solution of bee venom is injected. There is no consistency in the dosage forms sold. The therapy is moderately expensive. Most patients who start on this agent stop within six months because of discomfort, side effects, lack of benefit, or cost.

**Conclusion:** This therapy is not recommended because of lack of evidence of benefit and because of the side effects and the danger of allergic reaction.

*In the opinion of the Committee, this is not recommended for the treatment of MS.*

OCTACOSANOL

**Description:** A simple long-chain alcohol.

**Rationale:** The use of octacosanol is based on the idea that MS involves a disturbance in the incorporation of long-chain fatty acids into myelin lipids and the suggestion that the corresponding long-chain alcohols might stimulate this process and thus correct the problem or perhaps accelerate repair of damaged myelin.

**Evaluation:** Daily administration of octacosanol in several dozen people with MS is said to have led to continued improvement in two of three patients and remission of symptoms over a few days or weeks in about 10 percent of patients. The treatment is also said to arrest the unrelated disease ALS in 75 percent of patients, and claims have been made that octacosanol is effective in the treatment of muscular atrophy, myasthenia gravis, amyotonia congenita, several types of cerebral palsy, brain damage, poststroke syndrome, myositis (inflammation of voluntary muscle), dermatomyositis, and several other neuromuscular disorders. The findings depend on clinical impressions rather than quantified objective study. There has not been a controlled study, and the degree of improvement observed is comparable to that seen with treatments regarded as ineffective today.

**Risks/Costs:** Negligible.

**Conclusion:** There is no objective evidence at the present time that this treatment is of value in MS.

> *In the opinion of the Committee, there appears to be no generally accepted scientific basis for use of this therapy. It has never been tested in a properly controlled trial. Risks are undetermined.*

SUPEROXIDE DISMUTASE (ORGOTEIN, ORGOSEIN, PALOSEIN)

**Description:** Superoxide dismutase (SOD) is a metalloprotein enzyme that combines with and "neutralizes" free radicals of oxygen (superoxides) appearing as a normal toxic by-product of cellular metabolism. It is available in health food stores as an extract of liver in tablet form and is used in veterinary practice as an antiinflammatory agent (by injection).

**Rationale:** The theory has been developed that tissue superoxides may be involved in the "hardening" of connective tissue in some forms of chronic inflammation and in tissue degeneration and aging. There is evidence in both experimental allergic encephalomyelitis (EAE) and MS of increased generation of reactive oxygen species that may damage myelin. Administration of SOD has been shown to attenuate experimental inflammatory demyelination. Theoretically, augmenting the supply of SOD, which would be presumed to reduce the level of superoxides, would reduce inflammation and lessen these toxic effects.

**Evaluation:** SOD has been widely advertised as useful in a variety of inflammatory and sclerotic conditions. When injected, it has been shown to be safe and effective in reducing inflammation after irradiation and tissue damage of the joints, bladder, and bowel. There are unsubstantiated claims of its usefulness in rheumatoid arthritis and MS. Because proteins are denatured and digested in the stomach, it is doubtful that this substance would remain biologically active after oral use. In one uncontrolled trial of 23 MS patients, the results could not be differentiated from those expected in a placebo response. In a recent controlled, double-blind study of 200 patients given orgotein or placebo over the course of a year, with further observation for two years, no attempt was made to obtain objective data by scoring the severity of disease or counting the actual number of relapses; yet the claim was made that all treated patients improved, three-fourths of them resumed work, and flare-ups of MS were eliminated.

**Risks/Costs:** SOD apparently is not toxic.

**Conclusion:** From available reports, there appears to be no published evidence that SOD is effective in MS.

*In the opinion of the Committee, there appears to be some scientific basis for use of this therapy. It has, however, never been tested in a properly controlled trial. Risks are undetermined.*

### PROCAINE HYDROCHLORIDE

**Description:** Procaine is a simple chemical with anesthetic properties. KH3 is the proprietary name for a procaine compound in capsule form available by prescription in limited areas of the United States and in Europe. It is said to improve physical and mental efficiency and to improve the depression associated with old age.

**Rationale:** Procaine is used in local surgery and in skin creams for treatment of local burns (e.g., sunburn). There is no known basis for its use in the treatment of MS.

**Evaluation:** No evaluation of KH3 has been conducted for MS because there is no clinical indication for its use. Scattered anecdotal reports of treatment have led to clinical effects that cannot be differentiated from the placebo response.

**Risks/Costs:** The material is not approved for use by the FDA. There are no risks except in rare cases of procaine allergy.

**Conclusion:** There is no indication for the use of procaine in MS.

*In the opinion of the Committee, there appears to be no gen-
erally accepted scientific basis for use of this therapy. It has
never been tested in a properly controlled trial. Its use carries
significant risk.*

## Dimethyl Sulfoxide

**Description:** Dimethyl sulfoxide (DMSO) is a potent solvent for chemicals and has been widely used in industry as a degreaser.

**Rationale:** Because of its rapid absorption by the skin and its qualities as
a liniment, DMSO has been used for the treatment of sprains and muscle pains in animals. It is under study in purified form for oral or intravenous administration or administration by way of the skin to determine
whether it can help transport drugs more effectively into tissue cells for
treatment of specific diseases. In animal studies, it has been shown to be
immunosuppressive, and research is under way to determine its possible
usefulness in the treatment of autoimmune diseases. DMSO is approved
by the FDA for administration into the bladder in a 50% solution for
therapy of an uncommon intractable form of chronic inflammation.

**Evaluation:** DMSO has achieved some notoriety as a nonprescription
drug for the treatment of arthritis and other chronic debilitating diseases.
There is no evidence at this time that it provides a predictable change in
the clinical severity of any of these conditions beyond what can be
explained by the placebo response. There has been no controlled study of
DMSO in MS.

**Risks/Costs:** DMSO may cause cataracts. Its rapid rate of absorption carries the danger of absorbing toxic contaminants (if "industrial grade" is
used). Side effects include rashes, nausea, vomiting, chills, drowsiness,
and a characteristic garlic odor on the breath. DMSO is relatively inexpensive and is available as a nonprescription item in health food stores,
hardware stores, and various other outlets.

**Conclusion:** There is no acceptable medical evidence to support the use of
DMSO in MS at the present time. There are risks of serious side effects.

*In the opinion of the Committee, there appears to be no gen-
erally accepted scientific basis for use of this therapy. It has
never been tested in a properly controlled trial. There are risks
of serious side effects.*

### ALPHASAL (FORMERLY CHOLORAZONE OR VITAMIN X)

**Description:** A product of electrolysis of a saline solution. If used immediately, it contains ozone. Taken orally or by injection.

**Rationale:** This product was developed in Greece and has been recommended for prophylaxis or treatment of many diseases. The rationale for its use is obscure.

**Evaluation:** Only anecdotal information is available. More than 500 individuals with 50 different diseases are said to have been treated under the supervision of the inventor. Positive results were obtained in all 50 cases, and "cures" were reported in 30 patients, including those with MS, arthritis, and cancer. No controlled studies have been done.

**Risks/Costs:** Not known.

**Conclusion:** No scientifically acceptable evidence exists for the usefulness of alphasal in MS.

> *In the opinion of the Committee, there appears to be no generally accepted scientific basis for use of this therapy. It has never been tested in a properly controlled trial. Risks are undetermined.*

### CELLULAR THERAPY

**Description:** Injection of ground-up brain or other tissues freshly prepared from unborn calves, lambs, or pigs.

**Rationale:** A Swiss clinic developed this approach more than 40 years ago for the treatment of a wide variety of diseases. Injection of fetal tissue corresponding to the diseased tissue of the patient was theorized to bring new vigor and fight disease in that tissue. It is not regarded seriously as a scientific theory today.

**Evaluation:** Many patients with MS were treated with fetal brain. Improvement was claimed in the majority of patients on the basis of subjective impressions. No controlled studies were done.

**Risks/Costs:** Two cases were reported in which the injections produced autoimmunization, and the patients developed EAE comparable to the experimental disease in laboratory animals. One death resulting from this "treatment" has been reported.

**Conclusion:** What little published information is available suggests that this treatment should be considered ineffective in MS and potentially dangerous.

> *In the opinion of the Committee, there appears to be no generally accepted scientific basis for use of this therapy. It has never been tested in a properly controlled trial. Its use carries significant risk.*

ALLERGENS

**Description:** Repeated injections of food or other allergens; used in desensitization for asthma and hay fever.

**Rationale:** This treatment was based on the theory that MS might be an allergic reaction to common environmental substances.

**Evaluation:** There have been attempts to identify environmental allergens, including foods, that might play a role in the MS process. This was followed by attempts to affect the clinical course of MS by desensitization with increasing injections of the allergen. Elimination diets have also been tried. There is no convincing evidence that such allergies are more common in MS patients than in the general population or that these measures influenced the course of the disease.

**Risks/Costs:** Negligible risks. Cost of repeated injections is significant.

**Conclusion:** All available data suggest that this treatment should be considered ineffective in MS.

> *In the opinion of the Committee, there appears to be no generally accepted scientific basis for use of this therapy. It has never been tested in a properly controlled trial. It is relatively free of serious adverse side effects during long-term use. It is very expensive.*

RODILEMID

**Description:** A mixture of chelating (metal-binding) agents, developed in Rumania. It includes L-cysteine, the calcium sodium salt of ethylenediamine tetraacetic acid (EDTA), and calcium gluconate. It is taken as a series of six daily intramuscular injections at intervals of one to four months.

**Rationale:** This mixture was developed to "facilitate calcium penetration into the neuron" and thus "inhibit viral infection." It is said not to lower body or cell calcium and thus lacks the toxicity associated with chelation therapy. No studies have been done of the possible direct effects on nerve conduction or the antiinflammatory action on lymphocytes or macrophages.

**Evaluation:** In a long-term uncontrolled study, it was claimed that Rodilemid therapy gave lasting improvement (at least one point on the Kurtzke scale) in 80 percent of patients with chronic progressive or clinically stable MS. These results are unconfirmed thus far.

**Risks/Costs:** Toxicity appears to be low.

**Conclusion:** Rodilemid is unproven as a therapy for MS.

> *In the opinion of the Committee, there appears to be no generally accepted scientific basis for use of this therapy. It has never been tested in a properly controlled trial. Risks are undetermined.*

AUTOGENOUS VACCINE

**Description:** Vaccine prepared from bacteria growing in or on the patient's own body.

**Rationale:** Such vaccines were used half a century ago on the old theory that various diseases might be allergic reactions to the individual's own bacteria.

**Evaluation:** No controlled trials have been carried out in MS, and there is no accepted basis for such trials at present. Some reports indicate that the treatment is dangerous.

**Risks/Costs:** Not commercially available, and costs are undetermined.

**Conclusion:** Bacterial products may be interferon (IFN) inducers, including IFN-gamma. Because of this and the lack of controlled studies, this treatment should not be used.

> *In the opinion of the Committee, this therapy should not be used because of reported harmful effects.*

PRONEUT

**Description:** A combination of measles vaccine, influenza vaccine, and histamine phosphate, the dose being individually determined for each patient.

**Rationale:** Proneut is used experimentally as a type of "provocation therapy" or "provocation-neutralization therapy" in MS treatment, using three components suspected of being the causative agent in MS. The patient receives repeated subcutaneous doses of the mixture.

**Evaluation:** The use of Proneut has been limited to subjective observations in an uncontrolled series of MS patients, with no attempt at full neurologic evaluation. The results reported are compatible with a placebo effect.

**Risks/Costs:** A high fee is charged for a simple mixture, which patients are taught to self-administer.

**Conclusion:** There appears to be no convincing evidence at present that this treatment is effective in MS.

> *In the opinion of the Committee, there appears to be no generally accepted scientific basis for use of this therapy. It has never been tested in a properly controlled trial. Risks are undetermined. It is very expensive.*

ALPHA-FETOPROTEIN (α-FETOPROTEIN)

**Description:** Alpha-fetoprotein (AFP) is a protein produced by the liver of the fetus in the womb to protect it against the mother's immune system. It has been purified and used experimentally.

**Rationale:** The severity of MS sometimes diminishes during late pregnancy, when the fetus is producing large amounts of AFP. Experimentally, AFP is effective in suppressing EAE. It therefore may be of interest for a trial in MS.

**Evaluation:** A trial of AFP in MS is under consideration at the present time.

**Risks/Costs:** Not known.

**Conclusion:** None at present.

*In the opinion of the Committee, there appears to be no generally accepted scientific basis for use of this therapy. It has never been tested in a properly controlled trial. Risks are undetermined.*

IMMUNOBIOLOGICAL REVITALIZATION

**Description:** Purified rabbit antibodies against human bone marrow, spleen, and thymus, supplemented by an undefined "human placental product."

**Rationale:** A Russian scientist, Bogomoletz, originally described the use of antibody against lymphoid tissues (so-called "antireticulo-cytotoxic" antibody) as a stimulant to immune function when the antibody was given in repeated low doses.

**Evaluation:** This treatment was widely used in the former Soviet Union before World War II and has since spread to the rest of the world. As "immunobiological revitalization," it is said to cure diseases affecting all systems of the body, including allergies, cancer, and mental disease; improve sexuality; extend life span; and provide beneficial cosmetic effects. These claims have also been made for MS. Thirty-eight patients were treated between 1974 and 1979. No objective observations were made to substantiate the claim.

**Risks/Costs:** The treatment is usually offered as part of a broad and expensive "program." Risks are not known.

**Conclusion:** Based on the evidence examined, this treatment is not recommended.

*In the opinion of the Committee, there appears to be no generally accepted scientific basis for use of this therapy. It has never been tested in a properly controlled trial. Risks are undetermined. It is very expensive.*

PROTEOLYTIC ENZYMES

**Description:** A mixture of digestive enzymes (pancreatin, chymotrypsin, and several others); given intravenously in repeated doses.

**Rationale:** A mixture of proteolytic enzymes is reported to have therapeutic action in inflammatory diseases caused by immune complexes (antigen-antibody aggregates), such as glomerulonephritis and rheumatoid arthritis, as well as in coagulation disorders. Immune complex formation may possibly play a role in lesion formation in acute MS.

**Evaluation:** A standardized commercial system enzyme mixture has been used in 80 MS patients for more than five years in a preliminary study carried out in Austria. With early high-dose administration, acute attacks are reported to be aborted in some cases. With long-term treatment, it is claimed that further attacks and progression are prevented in 50 percent of patients. The treatment is relatively ineffective in patients already treated for some time with azathioprine, ACTH, or corticosteroids. Controlled studies are under way.

**Risks/Costs:** This therapy is said to be essentially nontoxic. However, any intravenous injection, especially with foreign proteins, carries substantial potential risks. The cost of repetitive intravenous therapy usually is high.

**Conclusion:** Inadequate published information exists to permit informed judgment about this therapy.

> *In the opinion of the Committee, there appears to be no generally accepted scientific basis for this therapy. It has never been tested in a properly controlled trial. Risks are undetermined.*

### Chelation Therapy with Ethylenediamine Tetraacetic Acid (EDTA)

**Description:** A simple chemical that chelates (binds) metals very efficiently and is used in cases of lead poisoning to remove lead from the body. Must be injected intravenously over several hours.

**Rationale:** Several practitioners have advocated the use of "chelation therapy" for MS, along with a wide variety of other diseases, including cancer, Parkinson's disease, arthritis, heart attacks, and strokes, as well as simpler problems such as leg cramps, poor vision, senility, poor memory, and so forth.

**Evaluation:** The FDA, the Veterans Administration, and other professional associations are unanimous in calling "chelation therapy" worthless for the purposes claimed. The Harvard Medical School *Health Letter* concludes: "There is no credible evidence that chelation therapy works as claimed . . . except as an elaborate placebo."

**Risks/Costs:** This "therapy" is "potentially" lethal without adequate supervision. It was implicated by federal officials in 14 deaths at one clinic. Costs may run as high as $6,000 for treatment extending over several months.

**Conclusion:** Chelation therapy for MS is not based on acceptable published evidence and is dangerous.

> *In the opinion of the Committee, there appears to be no generally accepted scientific basis for use of this therapy. It has never been tested in a properly controlled trial. Its use carries significant risk. It is very expensive.*

## Injected Materials and Oral Administration

### CALCIUM OROTATE, CALCIUM AMINOETHYL PHOSPHATE

**Description:** Calcium orotate and calcium aminoethyl phosphate (AEP) are calcium salts of synthetic organic compounds; given intravenously and by mouth.

**Rationale:** These substances were developed to facilitate the carrying of calcium and making it more available for body metabolism.

**Evaluation:** Both compounds have been used for over 20 years in a clinic in Germany for the treatment of conditions considered to be inflammatory or autoimmune in nature. The treatment, especially calcium AEP, is said to have a very favorable effect on 5 to 78 percent of patients with MS. Objective and quantified data are not available, and there is no documented proof that therapies of this sort produce any benefit. They are clearly the subject of considerable commercial exploitation.

**Risks/Costs:** There are said to be no significant side effects. Costs are high.

**Conclusion:** In the absence of a properly designed clinical study, the claim of favorable effect remains undocumented.

> *In the opinion of the Committee, there appears to be no generally accepted scientific basis for use of this therapy. It has never been tested in a properly controlled trial. It is relatively free of serious adverse side effects during long-term use. It is very expensive.*

SODIUM BICARBONATE, PHOSPHATES

**Description:** Simple chemicals; given intravenously (sodium bicarbonate) or by mouth (phosphates).

**Rationale:** Experimental studies suggested that nerve fiber conduction would be improved by decreasing the concentration of calcium available to demyelinated fibers.

**Evaluation:** In clinical trials, it has been possible to reduce calcium levels temporarily by giving intravenous sodium bicarbonate or large oral doses of phosphates, both of which bind calcium. These trials resulted in rapid but temporary measurable improvement in a number of neurologic defects. Continued use of such agents and long-term low calcium levels are not compatible with good health. Therefore, these agents are not satisfactory treatments for MS. The studies do demonstrate that nerve fiber conduction can be favorably altered by chemical means and encourage the search for agents that can be used over extended periods.

**Risks/Costs:** Long-term use is not compatible with good health.

**Conclusion:** These substances are not recommended as treatments.

> *In the opinion of the Committee, there appears to be no generally accepted scientific basis for use of this therapy. It has never been tested in a properly controlled trial. Risks are undetermined.*

## Oral Administration

ORAL CALCIUM + MAGNESIUM + VITAMIN D

**Description:** Inexpensive chemicals available commercially; taken by mouth.

**Rationale:** Epidemiologic studies suggested a correlation of MS prevalence with restricted intake of calcium, magnesium, and vitamin D. This observation is supported by the finding of abnormal calcium and magnesium levels in the serum of people with MS. Finally, deficiency is thought to produce instability of myelin because both minerals are essential to the myelination process.

**Evaluation:** In a small preliminary trial, patients were fed calcium, magnesium, and vitamin D for a period of one to two years. They experienced fewer relapses of MS during the period of treatment than would be expected from their histories. However, this observation is difficult to interpret because the frequency of relapses in individual patients tends to diminish with time. A larger, controlled study is being planned.

**Risks/Costs:** Inexpensive.

**Conclusion:** The efficacy of this treatment is as yet undocumented.

*In the opinion of the Committee, there appears to be no generally accepted scientific basis for use of this therapy. It has never been tested in a properly controlled trial. Risks are undetermined.*

ST. JOHN'S WORT

**Description:** A plant, the active ingredient of which is hypericum. It has been used for hundreds of years and recently has been popularized as a treatment for many conditions.

**Rationale:** It is thought to have some effect on the neurochemicals in the brain that are involved in mood and depression.

**Evaluation:** At present 23 trials, 15 of which were well designed and controlled, have shown some benefit in depression over the placebo group. It may be beneficial in mild depression, but standard antidepressants are recommended if depression is more severe. Many people who take St. John's wort do so because there are fewer side effects than many conventional antidepressants, but the treatment is only beneficial in mild depression and does have side effects, especially increasing sensitivity of the skin to sunlight (photosensitivity). Another concern is the variability of such unregulated medicines, and a study of 10 different brands showed that the recommended dose varied from 300 to 900 mg, some had no expiration dates, and three combined it with other products. A major study comparing St. John's wort with a selective serotonin reuptake inhibitor (SSRI) antidepressant and a placebo is under way.

**Risks/Costs:** Risks are uncertain if taken in recommended amounts. Inexpensive.

**Conclusion:** St. John's wort may be helpful in mild depression. Standard antidepressants should be used if depression is more severe or protracted.

*In the opinion of the Committee, St. John's wort is not a treatment for MS, but may be beneficial in patients who have mild depression or mood change.*

### HYPERIMMUNE COLOSTRUM (IMMUNE MILK)

**Description:** Pregnant cows are inoculated with measles vaccine or other viruses considered to be possibly related to MS. Colostrum (early milk), collected by veterinarians from these cows during the first two days after delivery, is frozen for preservation and subsequently taken by mouth.

**Rationale:** In humans, antibodies cross the placenta from the mother's circulation into the baby's circulation, providing it with immunity against a variety of infections before birth. In cattle, antibodies do not cross the placenta but pass from the mother to the newborn calf in the colostrum during nursing. The use of hyperimmune bovine colostrum as a treatment for MS is based on evidence that one or more viruses may be associated with the development of MS.

**Evaluation:** No studies have been done to determine whether there are antibodies to the vaccines used in the serum of the cows, in the colostrum, or in the patients. In general, bovine antibodies are not absorbed by adult humans from the stomach or intestine. A sizable number of people with MS in various parts of the United States have received hyperimmune bovine colostrum. The responses of patients were obtained by questionnaire, and a majority of patients reported improvement. However, much of the improvement related to stamina, well-being, pain, and activity level.

In a preliminary double-blind, cross-over study of 12 people with MS, three showed some worsening when taken off immune colostrum; two of these had very mild disease to start with.

In a pilot Japanese study that was published in 1984, most MS patients who were given immune colostrum containing measles antibody "improved," whereas most patients in a smaller group who were given normal colostrum worsened. No data are provided as to duration or severity of disease or the possible occurrence of exacerbations in individual patients, and there was no matching or randomization of test groups and control groups.

**Risks/Costs:** The cost of hyperimmune colostrum appears to be modest. A few people reported skin rash, mild allergic reaction, or "not feeling well."

**Conclusion:** This treatment remains unproven and is not recommended. A clinical trial of adequate size would be required to determine whether it has any value.

> *In the opinion of the Committee, there appears to be no generally accepted scientific basis for use of this therapy. It has never been tested in a properly controlled trial. Risks are undetermined.*

METABOLIC THERAPY

**Description:** A complex program of regimens and medications said to affect mineral balance, diet (both how much and what is in it), and bowel function (e.g., alkalinity of the small intestine); also immune colostrum and high doses of vitamin C (as "antiviral agents"), SOD, vitamin A, "thymotropic" tablets to "stimulate the immune system," octacosanol, and B complex vitamins.

**Rationale:** The components of this program are discussed individually elsewhere in this book.

**Evaluation:** "Metabolic therapy" has never been subjected to a scientifically planned clinical trial in which objective measurements of effect can be determined. As noted elsewhere in this book, the Committee is not aware of any scientific basis for any of the components of this program. Various forms of "metabolic therapy" have been advocated as cures for cancer and arthritis, with poor evidence of effectiveness.

**Risks/Costs:** Vitamins A and C in large doses produce toxic side effects. Costs are substantial.

**Conclusion:** This is an unproven, expensive, and possibly dangerous procedure with no known scientific basis.

> *In the opinion of the Committee, there appears to be no generally accepted scientific basis for use of this therapy. It has never been tested in a properly controlled trial. Long-term use may be associated with significant serious side effects. It is very expensive.*

PROMAZINE HYDROCHLORIDE (SPARINE)

**Description:** A phenothiazine drug.

**Rationale:** The hypothesis is offered that specific immune responses to acute viral infection are accompanied by blood–brain barrier damage. Drugs that antagonize a "pressor" effect during the prodromal phase that precedes exacerbations are thought to abort the disease process.

**Evaluation:** Evidence to support the use of Sparine is entirely anecdotal. No controlled trials have been carried out. Other drugs said to have similar effects, based on similar anecdotal grounds, include oxprenolol, propranolol, and Largactil.

**Risks/Costs:** Promazine can cause hypotension, and it may cause a parkinsonian syndrome with long-term use. It is inexpensive.

**Conclusion:** The value of phenothiazine and related drugs in aborting MS exacerbations is unsubstantiated.

> *In the opinion of the Committee, there appears to be no generally accepted scientific basis for use of this therapy. It has never been tested in a properly controlled trial. Long-term use may be associated with significant serious side effects.*

## LE GAC THERAPY

**Description:** Treatment with broad-spectrum antibiotics (Terramycin, tetracycline) combined with hot baths.

**Rationale:** MS is attributed to infection with rickettsiae, infectious agents intermediate between bacteria and viruses. In one study, antibodies to rickettsiae were found more frequently in people with MS than in a series of controls, an observation that has been repeatedly suggested and just as often refuted since 1913. Use of broad-spectrum antibiotics is intended to cure such infection.

**Evaluation:** No convincing epidemiologic or bacteriologic evidence to relate MS to rickettsial infection has ever been obtained. People with MS show more frequent and higher antibody levels to a variety of infectious agents than do controls, probably as a consequence of faulty immune regulation. Le Gac therapy has been supported by a series of anecdotal cases in which patients, usually treated during an acute attack of MS, subsequently improved. No controlled trial of the therapy has ever been done.

**Risks/Costs:** Negligible. Hot baths usually cause transient worsening of symptoms.

**Conclusion:** Based on evidence examined, this treatment is not recommended.

*In the opinion of the Committee, there appears to be no generally accepted scientific basis for use of this therapy. It has never been tested in a properly controlled trial. Its use carries significant risk.*

### NYSTATIN

**Description:** An antifungal agent that is particularly effective against yeast infections (*Candida albicans*); usually employed with a yeast-free, low-carbohydrate diet.

**Rationale:** Two physicians have tried to relate a variety of chronic disorders to overgrowth of *Candida albicans* in the intestinal tract after use of carbohydrate-rich diets, birth control pills, steroids, or other antibiotics. MS is included, along with schizophrenia, depression, psoriasis, arthritis, headache, premenstrual tension, and various other nervous system disorders.

**Evaluation:** There is no widely accepted scientific or medical evidence that any of the aforementioned conditions are related to candidiasis. Evidence for efficacy of nystatin in MS is largely anecdotal. Rigorous controlled studies have not been reported.

**Risks/Costs:** Modest.

**Conclusion:** Use of nystatin in MS is not recommended.

*In the opinion of the Committee, there appears to be no generally accepted scientific basis for use of this therapy. It has never been tested in a properly controlled trial. It is relatively free of serious adverse side effects during short-term use.*

## Physical and Surgical Manipulations

### ACUPUNCTURE, ACUPRESSURE, QIGONG

**Description:** These procedures are part of traditional Chinese medicine (TCM). Acupuncture is a 4,000-year-old Chinese procedure that has been known to the Western world since the 1600s. It is performed by inserting fine needles into specific skin sites with the expectation of influencing the function of underlying organs. The belief is that body energy flows in channels (meridians) that connect to organs and an imbalance can be restored by the acupuncture needles inserted into 365 points (corresponding to the days in the year, although over the centuries up to 2,000 points have been identified). Twirling, vibrating, or electrically stimulating the needles is considered to enhance the effectiveness of the procedure. A variation on this approach is the use of acupressure over the same points. Qigong is an approach to restore balance by deep breathing, concentration, and relaxation exercises. Some Qigong masters claim to have healing energies released from their fingertips. TCM also uses pulse diagnosis, identifying more than 25 pulse qualities, such as "soggy" and "tight."

**Rationale:** Acupuncture has been used extensively for the relief of pain of various origins. It appears to be associated with increased endorphin activity [natural morphine-like substances in the central nervous system (CNS)]. The use of acupuncture might be beneficial for relief of pain and muscle spasm.

**Evaluation:** There is anecdotal evidence that some patients treated with acupuncture have lessening of pain. There is no evidence that progression of MS or of any other disease is altered by acupuncture.

**Risks/Costs:** Any procedure that involves penetration of the skin by needles may carry the risk of hepatitis. Studies of acupuncture have reported fainting, lung puncture, increased pain, and other adverse reactions. Costs are moderately high for repeated long-term treatments.

**Conclusion:** Based on the evidence examined, this treatment is considered to have no effect on the disease process in MS and has not been shown to have any value in the symptomatic management of patients with disease. Some patients may experience temporary relief of pain.

*In the opinion of the Committee, there appears to be no generally accepted scientific basis for use of this therapy in MS. It may be helpful in reducing pain. It is moderately expensive for long-term therapy.*

DORSAL COLUMN STIMULATION

**Description:** The dorsal columns of the spinal cord are large bundles of nerve fibers that carry the sense of touch and the sense of position from the legs, trunk, and arms to the brain. The spinal cord is protected by a connective tissue wrapping known as dura. Electrical stimulation of the dorsal columns requires implantation of two electrodes on the overlying dura. This formerly necessitated an open operation but is now done by passing the electrodes through a special needle. The electrodes are connected with an implanted stimulator or radio receiver.

**Rationale:** The use of dorsal column stimulation (DCS) in MS began empirically when the procedure was used with an MS patient to control pain and it was noted that the patient functioned better after sessions of stimulation. Subsequently, it was claimed that DCS favorably altered the functioning of the neural circuits of the CNS, especially the spinal cord and brain stem, and produced measurable changes in evoked potentials and in both subjective state and objective neurologic function in some patients.

**Evaluation:** Claims are made of benefit from DCS in a variety of diseases. These include athetosis, cerebral palsy, dystonia, posttraumatic and post-stroke spasticity, epilepsy, and "degenerative disease." In one series of 300 such cases, 70 to 85 percent of patients were said to have shown improvement in one or another neural function. However, in at least four series of MS patients in which there was careful neurologic follow-up, a few patients showed initial subjective improvement, but none showed either subjective or objective benefit at the end of two years and most had abandoned the treatment.

**Risks/Costs:** Infection, hemorrhage, and serious spinal cord injury have occurred in a small proportion of patients. Slipping of electrodes out of place or breakage of electrode wires occurs in up to 65 percent of cases. This requires surgery to replace or remove the electrodes. In a small proportion of cases, the operation may be complicated by hemorrhage at the operative site, spinal cord compression, and paraplegia (total paralysis) of the lower limbs. The costs include surgical fees, operating room costs, and hospitalization, which may amount to more than $25,000 and usually are not reimbursable by third-party carriers.

**Conclusion:** This procedure is ineffective and dangerous. The costs and the risks are high. It is not recommended for use in people with MS.

> *In the opinion of the Committee, this therapy should not be used because of reported harmful effects. Its use carries significant risk. It is very expensive.*

HYPERBARIC OXYGEN

**Description:** Breathing oxygen under increased pressure in a specially constructed chamber.

**Rationale:** Hyperbaric oxygen (HBO) has been used effectively in burns, gas gangrene, and air embolism. It has been reported to improve mental function in elderly patients. Early reports suggested that HBO might produce temporary improvement in people with MS. HBO is also immunosuppressive and suppresses EAE, the animal model of MS. However, oxygen at normal pressure is also reported to suppress EAE.

**Evaluation:** HBO has been used over several years in the treatment of a considerable number of MS patients in the United States, the United Kingdom, Italy, and the former Soviet Union. In uncontrolled studies and one controlled study, patients with chronic progressive disease were reported to show significant improvement after a course of treatment lasting several weeks. The results of six separate, controlled, double-blind studies were reported, which mimicked in detail the techniques described earlier as effective, including (in one instance) monthly booster treatments extending over six months. Assessments made use of magnetic resonance imaging (MRI) and electrophysiologic techniques in addition to more conventional neurologic and laboratory procedures. These trials, which were carried out in the United States, the United Kingdom, Canada, and the Netherlands, unanimously demonstrated that HBO is without effect on any objective parameter of the disease process, with the single exception of minimal bladder improvement in some patients.

**Risks/Costs:** The procedure entails high cost because the equipment is expensive, skilled technicians are required, and frequent repeated visits are necessary. Exposure to oxygen at higher pressures or for longer periods than those recommended may produce serious side effects in the nervous system, the most extreme being blindness or convulsive episodes. Such effects may be seen in a small percentage of patients even when they are correctly treated.

**Conclusion:** Large-scale, double-blind, controlled studies have proven that HBO is ineffective as a treatment for MS.

*In the opinion of the Committee, this therapy has been adequately tested and shown to be without value. Its use carries significant risk. It is very expensive.*

### TRANSCUTANEOUS NERVE STIMULATION

**Description:** Transcutaneous nerve stimulation (TNS) is a procedure in which electrodes are placed on the surface of the skin over certain nerves and electrical stimulation is carried out. The dose, which is varied by changing frequency, pulse width, and intensity (amplitude), determines which nerve fibers are activated.

**Rationale:** The stimulation of the CNS from the periphery is thought to improve CNS performance generally. This is actually a variant of acupuncture technique, and in some ways it resembles old-fashioned "counterirritant" techniques (mustard plaster, etc.). The newest way of doing the same thing is with the use of a low-powered laser beam. Stimulation for 20 to 30 minutes gives objective pain relief, and this has been clearly related to release of morphine-like compounds within the CNS and cerebrospinal fluid (CSF). TNS is sometimes used in conjunction with oral administration of the unnatural amino acid d-phenylalanine, which is claimed to have an endorphin (morphine-like) effect, and vitamin Bl2.

**Evaluation:** Subjective improvement and reduced spasticity have been reported to an extent not seen in MS patients subjected to sham stimulation. TNS is also said to reduce cerebellar tremor. Insufficient information exists to permit evaluation of this "treatment" because quantitative objective data have not been reported so far.

**Risks/Costs:** Local skin irritation under an electrode may occur. Some patients with dysesthesias complain that their discomfort is increased by TNS. TNS does not have the drawbacks of invasive DCS.

**Conclusion:** TNS is a moderately effective treatment for pain, but there is no evidence that it alters the underlying disease in MS.

> *In the opinion of the Committee, there appears to be no generally accepted scientific basis for use of this therapy in the treatment of MS. It may be helpful in symptomatic management. It is relatively free of serious adverse side effects during long-term use.*

### THALAMOTOMY, THALAMIC STIMULATION

**Description:** Destruction of part of the thalamus by surgical means. More recently, electrical stimulation of the thalamus by surgically implanted electrodes has been reported to have a similar effect.

**Rationale:** The thalamus is a central region in the upper part of the brain that contributes to the control of movement. Tremor and certain other involuntary movements can be reduced or abolished by thalamotomy or thalamic stimulation, and this procedure is used in various neurologic diseases.

**Evaluation:** Loss of coordination in MS is often associated with tremor during use of the arms or legs. In patients with severe tremors, thalamotomy has been performed with relief of the tremor but without effect on other neurologic defects. Patients who had tremor for at least one year were selected to be certain that it would not remit spontaneously. Tremor frequently recurs within a few years after the operation. Surgeons currently are turning away from thalamotomy because of the attendant risks and implanting electrodes in the same part of the brain as a less dangerous means of controlling tremor. There also is evidence that demyelination can develop along the areas of the brain through which the instruments passed.

**Risks/Costs:** The risks are those of complications attending any brain operation. Thalamotomy on one side may result in weakness of the arm and leg on the opposite side, disturbance of recent memory, or speech and language disturbance; these may be due to enlargement of the operative wound by bleeding, especially in patients with high blood pressure. There also may be exacerbation of the MS. Although unilateral thalamic lesions carry a modest risk, there is always a chance that MS will have damaged the other side of the thalamus. The risk of serious disability is high under such circumstances. Bilateral thalamotomy frequently causes pseudobulbar palsy and results in severe speech and swallowing difficulties. Costs, including surgeon's fees, operating room charges, and hospitalization, are very high.

**Conclusion:** Based on the evidence examined, thalamotomy and thalamic stimulation are not recommended for MS except in a small number of carefully selected MS patients, and even there the beneficial effect is of limited duration and is associated with substantial risks.

*In the opinion of the Committee, this therapy is not recommended but might be considered in patients with incapacitating tremor. Its use carries significant risk. It is very expensive.*

## SYMPATHECTOMY AND GANGLIONECTOMY

**Description:** Sympathetic nerves and ganglions supplying blood vessels to the head are surgically removed in an effort to increase blood supply to the CNS.

**Rationale:** A division of the nervous system called the autonomic nervous system controls such bodily functions as intestinal motility, heart rate, blood pressure, and blood vessel tone. Its sympathetic component constricts blood vessels, while parasympathetic activity dilates them. The use of this technique is based on the scientifically unproven assumption that the MS process involves inadequate local blood supply in the brain and spinal cord.

**Evaluation:** In the past, numerous agents intended to affect blood vessels and blood supply to the nervous system have been tried in MS treatment, but all have been abandoned as ineffective. The reported results of sympathectomy also were inconclusive.

**Risks/Costs:** Those associated with major surgery.

**Conclusion:** There is no convincing evidence that this surgical procedure is effective in treating MS.

> *In the opinion of the Committee, there appears to be no generally accepted scientific basis for use of this therapy. It has never been tested in a properly controlled trial. Its use carries significant risk. It is very expensive.*

## SURGICAL SPINAL CORD RELAXATION (CERVICOLORDODESIS)

**Description:** Surgical procedure to fix the cervical spine (in the neck) to restrict forward bending.

**Rationale:** It is suggested that the hard MS scar in parts of the spine subject to extreme motion, (e.g., the neck) tends to restrict the normal "viscoelastic flow" of the tissue (i.e., its free movement) and brings abnormal pressure to bear on nerve fibers in this part of the cord. Surgical restriction of neck movement would prevent this.

**Evaluation:** This procedure is alleged to be helpful in MS, but no data have been provided.

**Risks/Costs:** Both are high.

**Conclusion:** This therapy is without value in MS.

*In the opinion of the Committee, there appears to be no generally accepted scientific basis for use of this therapy. It has never been tested in a properly controlled trial. Its use carries significant risk. It is very expensive.*

VERTEBRAL ARTERY SURGERY

**Description:** An operation devised to eliminate kinking or narrowing of the vertebral arteries in the neck.

**Rationale:** The two vertebral arteries take their origin low in the neck and pass upward and backward, entering the skull along with the spinal cord. They join to form the basilar artery on the underside of the brain stem. The vertebral-basilar artery system provides most or all of the blood supply to the brain stem, cerebellum, and part of the cerebrum. It has been proposed that abnormality of the vertebral vessels causes hypoxia to the spinal cord and that correcting the narrowing surgically would improve blood flow.

**Evaluation:** There was a report of nine people with MS who benefited from the procedure in the 1970s, but details that would allow careful assessment were missing. The logic would seem to be flawed because many of the MS lesions are not in the distribution of the vertebral vascular system. This and other methods of treating MS by increasing blood flow have been abandoned.

**Conclusion:** The existing evidence does not support the conclusion that these procedures may be effective in the treatment of MS.

*In the opinion of the Committee, there appears to be no generally accepted scientific basis for use of this therapy. It has never been tested in a properly controlled trial. Its use carries significant risk. It is very expensive.*

ULTRASOUND

**Description:** Repeated application of ultrasound (i.e., high-frequency sound) to the area of the back next to the spinal column (backbone).

**Rationale:** Ultrasound, which permits physicians to probe certain parts of the body without harming the area probed, has great value as a diagnostic tool. It is sometimes used to reduce pain and spasm in muscles. In patients with MS, it is claimed that ultrasound "treatment" promotes the flow of lymph in lymph vessels draining the spinal cord and thus affects the disease process.

**Evaluation:** The use of ultrasound in MS has been stressed by certain clinicians in Austria. No controlled studies have been published, and reports of its effectiveness reflect mainly clinical impressions rather than objective observations. It is unclear how a treatment directed to the spinal cord could affect lesions in the brain. As noted earlier, a variety of treatments directed to improving blood and lymph flow in the CNS have been tried over many years and were judged ineffective.

**Risks/Costs:** Cost of repeated treatment is high.

**Conclusion:** The evidence suggests that this treatment is unlikely to be effective in MS. The high price clearly reflects commercial exploitation.

*In the opinion of the Committee, there appears to be no generally accepted scientific basis for use of this therapy. It has never been tested in a properly controlled trial. Risks are undetermined. It is very expensive.*

MAGNETOTHERAPY

**Description:** Repeated application of a low-frequency pulsing magnetic field. The strength of the field and the duration and frequency of exposure can be varied. Fifteen daily exposures at 2 to 10 H and less than 50 × 10–4 T are often used.

**Rationale:** Among many theories, a pulsing magnetic field is thought to improve cell functions, circulation, and oxygenation, as well as to reduce edema, inflammation, and scarring. Perhaps of more significance, it acts as the equivalent of repetitive high-frequency electrical stimulation of nerve fibers exposed to the field. Magnetism has been periodically revived and rejected as a treatment for a variety of condition over the last two centuries.

**Evaluation:** It has been claimed to be of value in both MS and a variety of other illnesses. A controlled clinical trial of magnetotherapy has been carried out in one center in Hungary. Nine of 10 patients with chronic stabilized disease showed mild to moderate improvement in spasticity (and accompanying pain), and half were reported to show improvement in cerebellar and bladder functions, whereas only 2 of 10 patients given a placebo exposure improved. Improvement was maintained over 4 to 16 weeks, with a slow return to pretreatment status. Reexposure resulted again in improvement. The treatment was effective when applied to the earlier placebo group in 8 of 10 patients. Results of an uncontrolled open study of 104 patients agreed with those obtained in the controlled study.

**Risks/Costs:** Not known. Expensive.

**Conclusion:** This treatment is not yet proven. Further controlled studies are under way.

> *In the opinion of the Committee, there appears to be no generally accepted scientific basis for use of this therapy. It has never been tested in a properly controlled trial. Risks are undetermined.*

## DENTAL OCCLUSAL THERAPY

**Description:** Correction of dental malocclusion with occlusal splints and other procedures, attention to other dental needs, and physical therapy to the muscles and structures of the temporomandibular joints. This approach is often coupled with a recommendation for a diet that is low in animal fat, with increased oil intake, vitamin and mineral supplements, and avoidance of refined foods (especially sugars).

**Rationale:** Dental malocclusions may be associated with dental distress, especially in the muscles and structures of the temporomandibular joints, and supposedly with decreased stress resistance in certain systemic muscle groups. The affected joints and muscles produce a continuing sensory input to the brain that is thought to result in decreased neurologic output and demyelination.

**Evaluation:** There is no known scientific basis for the claim that alterations in sensory input can affect the integrity of myelin. It is improbable that dental distress plays any role in the development of MS.

**Risks/Costs:** Dental procedures can be expensive.

**Conclusion:** There is neither scientific basis nor acceptable medical evidence that dental occulusion therapy could favorably influence the MS disease process.

*In the opinion of the Committee, there appears to be no generally accepted scientific basis for use of this therapy. It has never been tested in a properly controlled trial. It is relatively free of serious adverse side effects during long-term use. It is very expensive.*

REPLACEMENT OF MERCURY AMALGAM FILLINGS

**Description:** Removal and replacement of all fillings made of silver and mercury amalgam.

**Rationale:** This procedure, or even the removal of filled teeth, is based on the unsubstantiated claim that mercury leaks from amalgam fillings and damages the immune system, causing a broad range of problems, said to include MS and leukemia. Another theory suggests that the leaking mercury combines with nerve in the root canal and induces autoimmunization.

**Evaluation:** There is no sound epidemiologic evidence to relate MS to dental work. There is no evidence that MS patients have mercury levels higher than those of the normal population.

**Risks/Costs:** The risks are those of any dental procedures. It is very expensive.

**Conclusion:** There is no evidence to suggest that this procedure is of value in MS.

*In the opinion of the Committee, there appears to be no generally accepted scientific basis for use of this therapy. It has never been tested in a properly controlled trial. It is relatively free of serious adverse side effects during long-term use. It is very expensive.*

IMPLANTATION OF BRAIN SUBSTANCES

**Description:** Surgical implantation of pig brain in the abdominal wall.

**Rationale:** There is no clear rationale for this procedure.

**Evaluation:** Implantation of foreign tissue (as in cellular therapy) is a recurring theme in medicine. The newest variation on this theme is implantation of pig brain in MS patients. According to newspaper accounts, 13 of 15 patients reported symptomatic improvement within 24 hours. A critique by the German Multiple Sclerosis Society pointed out the absence of a scientific rationale for this procedure and its many dangers. The claimed results are regarded as a placebo effect.

**Risks/Costs:** The procedure is expensive and carries the usual risks of surgery, particularly infection and abscess formation at the implantation site, where the pig tissue undergoes rejection as a foreign graft. Such brain grafts also carry the risk of inducing autoimmune brain disease resembling the animal model EAE or transmitting pig viruses to the "treated" patient. By February 1982, 2 of 38 MS patients treated with this procedure in Germany had developed severe complications and 1 patient had died.

**Conclusion:** The evidence examined demonstrates that this treatment should be regarded as ineffective and dangerous.

*In the opinion of the Committee, this therapy should not be used because of reported harmful effects.*

HYSTERECTOMY

**Description:** Surgical removal of the uterus.

**Rationale:** It is suggested that progesterone can induce autoimmunization. It is then said to form immune complexes with antiprogesterone antibody, and these can damage various targeted tissues, among them the central and peripheral nervous systems. The lesions may manifest edema, inflammation, and tissue necrosis. They may mimic MS in the CNS.

**Evaluation:** Alleged to benefit MS. No data are provided to support this claim.

**Risks/Costs:** Risk is that of major surgery. Cost is high.

**Conclusion:** This procedure is not recommended for MS.

*In the opinion of the Committee, there appears to be no generally accepted scientific basis for use of this therapy and would constitute unnecessary surgery. It has never been tested in a properly controlled trial. It is very expensive.*

## Diet

### ALLERGEN-FREE DIET

**Description:** Regular use of a diet that eliminates foods that are known to produce hives, other skin eruptions, asthmatic attacks, and so on.

**Rationale:** This diet is based on the theory that the lesions of MS might be some sort of allergic reaction to common allergens from the environment.

**Evaluation:** The theory that MS might be due to an environmental allergy was popular in the late 1940s and early 1950s even though such allergies are not more common in MS patients than in the general population. Allergen-free diets were once used but are seldom used any longer.

**Risks/Costs:** Short-term use of the allergen-free diet has no associated risk. Inexpensive.

**Conclusion:** There is no demonstrated relationship between MS and external allergens. The diet has not been shown to be effective and has dropped out of favor. The necessary controlled studies have not been done.

> *In the opinion of the Committee, there appears to be no generally accepted scientific basis for use of this therapy. It has never been tested in a properly controlled trial. It is relatively free of serious adverse side effects during long-term use.*

### KOUSMINE DIET

**Description:** A low-fat, low-concentrated sugar, high-fiber diet, supplemented by vitamins A, C, D, E, and B complex.

**Rationale:** In a book entitled *Multiple Sclerosis Is Curable*, Dr. Catherine Kousmine, a Swiss physician, claims to have diagnosed and cured 55 patients. Her contention is that MS occurs as the result of an unhealthy diet. She suggests that the diet be started with a period of two to three days during which one eats only small quantities of raw fruit. One should then avoid all meats for two to three months.

**Evaluation:** There is no credible evidence that MS is caused by poor diet or dietary deficiencies. There are no properly controlled studies to prove efficacy of the diet. A low-fat, high-fiber diet with adequate nutritional balance is widely recommended for most people.

**Risks/Costs:** Risks are negligible.

**Conclusion:** There is no scientific evidence that this particular dietary method is effective in treating MS, although a low-fat healthy diet is recommended for most people.

> *In the opinion of the Committee, there appears to be no generally accepted scientific basis for use of this therapy, and it has never been tested in a properly controlled trial.*

GLUTEN-FREE DIET

**Description:** A balanced diet that excludes wheat and rye.

**Rationale:** The theory behind this approach suggests that the incidence of MS is high in areas of the world that raise and consume wheat and rye, which are gluten-containing grains, and low in areas that consume rice and corn, which do not contain gluten.

**Evaluation:** A balanced diet that excludes wheat and rye was suggested for use by people with MS. Subsequently, a diet was publicized that eliminated gluten and restricted carbohydrates, coffee, and alcohol. A two-year uncontrolled study of a gluten-free diet reported that both relapses and progression occurred in patients on the diet. However, the number of relapses and degree of progression could be readily explained by the natural course of MS. A small double-blind study (28 patients) showed no evidence of benefit from the diet.

**Risks/Costs:** Elimination of wheat and rye from the diet may result in inadequate protein intake unless protein is provided from other sources.

**Conclusion:** On the basis of the available data, this diet must be considered ineffective in MS.

> *In the opinion of the Committee, there appears to be no generally accepted scientific basis for use of this therapy. It has never been tested in a properly controlled trial. It is relatively free of serious adverse side effects during long-term use if adequate sources of protein are available in the diet.*

RAW FOOD, EVERS DIET

**Description:** A diet that contains only natural (unprocessed) foods, including a daily intake of germinated wheat.

**Rationale:** Dr. Joseph Evers, a German physician, believed that many illnesses were due to unnatural methods of production and processing of foods. His diet recommended the use of raw root vegetables, whole wheat bread, cheese, raw milk, raw eggs, butter, honey, and raw ham. Natural wine and brandy were permitted. Salt, sugar, confections, and condiments were forbidden. Also forbidden were leafy greens, stalks, and certain vegetables (salad greens, rhubarb, asparagus, cauliflower).

**Evaluation:** Although the Evers diet has been used by some people with MS, there is no evidence from the results that it affects the natural course of the disease. There also would seem to be no scientific basis for the claim that processed foods are chemically different from natural foods. None of the common food additives have been shown to produce lesions resembling those of MS.

**Risks/Costs:** There are no significant risks. Many so-called natural foods are expensive.

**Conclusion:** On the basis of existing information, it appears that this diet should be considered ineffective in MS.

> *In the opinion of the Committee, there appears to be no generally accepted scientific basis for use of this therapy. It has never been tested in a properly controlled trial. It is relatively free of serious adverse side effects during long-term use.*

### MacDougal Diet

**Description:** This diet combines a low-fat diet with a gluten-free diet and adds supplements of vitamins and minerals.

**Rationale:** The proponent of the diet, Professor Roger MacDougal, a writer and dramatist, believed that the combination diet was responsible for the almost complete disappearance of his MS symptoms.

**Evaluation:** There has been no scientific evidence that the MacDougal diet affects the natural course of MS.

**Risks/Costs:** Risks are negligible.

**Conclusion:** There appears to be no scientific evidence that this diet is effective in MS.

*In the opinion of the Committee, there appears to be no generally accepted scientific basis for use of this therapy. It has never been tested in a properly controlled trial. It is relatively free of serious adverse side effects during long-term use.*

## PECTIN- AND FRUCTOSE-RESTRICTED DIET
## (BASED ON METHANOL HYPOTHESIS)

**Description:** A diet from which unripe fruits, fruit juices, and pectin-containing fruits and vegetables are eliminated, supplemented with menadione (vitamin K3).

**Rationale:** A treatment based on the hypothesis that methanol (wood alcohol) produced by the metabolism of pectins (complex sugars) is converted to formaldehyde, which can bind to myelin components and lead to autoimmunization and consequent tissue damage. This process is thought to be exaggerated by ingestion of sugars that contain fructose, which is said to block the breakdown of formaldehyde, and pectins, which may contain some methanol. Menadione promotes the formation of tissue components (sphingomyelin), which may antagonize the methanol effect.

**Evaluation:** In a sizable uncontrolled series of MS patients on this diet, followed up for more than a year, relapses and exacerbations occurred, and a significant number deteriorated while on the diet. Approximately one-third of the patients dropped out of the trial. In the absence of controls, it is impossible to judge whether there was some reduction in progression or attacks. However, the results were similar to those obtained with other unproven therapies.

**Risks/Costs:** It is difficult and time-consuming to instruct patients in the use of the diet. Inexpensive.

**Conclusion:** The methanol hypothesis and the dietary regimen based on it remain unproven.

*In the opinion of the Committee, there appears to be no generally accepted scientific basis for use of this therapy. It has never been tested in a properly controlled trial. It is relatively free of serious adverse side effects during long-term use.*

## "Cambridge" and Other Liquid Diets

**Description:** A balanced, very low-calorie liquid that is used in treatment of obesity. Caloric intake is 330/day, with a suboptimal level of protein at 22 g/day. Extra potassium is supplied.

**Rationale:** Studies have shown no acceptable rationale for use of this diet in MS except to correct obesity.

**Evaluation:** Intense crash diets may lead to potassium deficiency, and several cases of sudden death resulting from such deficiency have been reported. The diet should only be undertaken with medical or other professional supervision.

**Risks/Costs:** Its use carries significant risks.

**Conclusion:** Based on the evidence examined, this diet is not recommended for treatment of MS.

> *In the opinion of the Committee, there appears to be no generally accepted scientific basis for use of this therapy. It has never been tested in a properly controlled trial. Its use carries significant risk.*

## Sucrose- and Tobacco-Free Diet

**Description:** Elimination of all food products that contain sucrose in the form of cane sugar, brown sugar, or maple sugar; molasses; sorghum; or dates; also products containing propylene glycol or glycol stearate (in shampoos). Tobacco is not to be used in any form.

**Rationale:** The diet is based on the belief that MS is caused by a form of allergy to sucrose or tobacco, as well as to the food additive propylene glycol. Glycol distearate, a constituent of many shampoos, is also incriminated.

**Evaluation:** The recommendation is based on personal experiences of eight MS patients with elimination diets of the type recommended. The diet is said to be ineffective in patients older than 50 years. No controlled study has been carried out.

**Risks/Costs:** Inexpensive.

**Conclusion:** This therapy remains unproven.

*In the opinion of the Committee, there appears to be no generally accepted scientific basis for use of this therapy. It has never been tested in a properly controlled trial. It is relatively free of serious adverse side effects during long-term use.*

## VITAMINS

**Description:** Individual vitamins or combinations of vitamins are taken in capsule or liquid form as a supplement to a normal diet.

**Rationale:** This approach assumes that MS may result from an unidentified vitamin deficiency.

**Evaluation:** Beginning in the late 1920s and continuing into the 1960s, there have been reports in the scientific literature of the use of vitamins in the treatment of MS. Various vitamins have been used alone or in a variety of combinations. Vitamins have been given orally (by mouth), parenterally (by injection), and intraspinally. Vitamin preparations used have included thiamine (B1), nicotinic acid (niacin), vitamin B12 (cyanocobalamin), ascorbic acid (vitamin C), tocopherol (vitamin E); liver therapy also has been used. Specific combinations of vitamins used have included fat-soluble vitamins (A, D, E, and K) with ammonium chloride, thiamine, and nicotinic acid. Improvement has been reported to occur in from 0 percent of patients in some studies up to 100 percent in others. None of the studies were subjected to the criteria and controls now used in the scientific evaluation of therapies for MS.

**Risks/Costs:** There is no evidence in animal experiments that vitamin deficiency produces lesions resembling those of MS. Vitamins A and D in high doses are toxic. Vitamin E and K in high doses can cause side effects. Moderately expensive depending on dosage and form. Supplementation with vitamins adds significantly to the cost of a normal balanced diet.

**Conclusion:** Adequate intake of vitamins is advised in all patients with MS, but there appears to be no scientific proof that supplementary doses of vitamins, alone or in combination, favorably affect the course of the disease.

*In the opinion of the Committee, there appears to be no generally accepted scientific basis for use of this therapy. It has never been tested in a properly controlled trial. Long-term use of high-dose vitamins may be associated with significant serious side effects.*

## MEGAVITAMIN THERAPY

**Description:** Massive doses of vitamins.

**Rationale:** As with other vitamin supplementation, large doses are used to make up for a presumed deficiency in uptake or utilization of one or more vitamins.

**Evaluation:** Megavitamin therapy has been used in the past in Canada and in a few localities in the United States. Although proponents have suggested that such therapy is effective in the treatment of MS, the reports are anecdotal and the Multiple Sclerosis Society of Canada stated that there is "no reliable scientific evidence to indicate that megavitamin therapy in any way influences the course of the disease."

**Risks/Costs:** It should be noted that excessive doses of some vitamins, especially A, D, E and K, can produce toxic effects. When pyridoxine (vitamin B6) is used in high doses, it sometimes produces disease of the peripheral nervous system, with weakness and loss of balance. This is especially a problem in patients who are already weak. Large doses of vitamins are expensive.

**Conclusion:** There appears to be no reliable evidence that megavitamin therapy influences the course of MS.

*In the opinion of the Committee, there appears to be no generally accepted scientific basis for use of this therapy. It has never been tested in a properly controlled trial. Long-term use may be associated with significant serious side effects.*

## MEGASCORBIC THERAPY

**Description:** Massive doses of vitamin C (ascorbic acid); referred to as an "orthomolecular" treatment.

**Rationale:** The claim is made that many people have a defective gene governing the liver enzymes concerned with carbohydrate metabolism. The consequent defect in vitamin C production, which is identified by a failure of spillover of this vitamin in the urine, results in "hypoascorbemia" and "chronic subclinical scurvy." This, in turn, is considered to underlie MS and a variety of other diseases, among them cancer, heart disease, stroke, arthritis, leukemia, diabetes, infectious diseases, and "many others." In the case of MS, high vitamin C levels are said to promote the patient's ability to produce interferon and resist viral infection.

**Evaluation:** The many diseases for which this therapy is proposed are unrelated to each other, and none has any known relation to vitamin C. The Committee believes that no scientifically adequate trial of this vitamin at megadose levels in MS has ever been carried out.

**Risks/Costs:** Continued treatment with vitamin C at the suggested levels is very expensive. Medical evidence has shown that high levels of ascorbic acid intake can produce stomach problems and kidney stones.

**Conclusion:** The value of megascorbic therapy in MS is unproven, and this treatment is not recommended.

*In the opinion of the Committee, there appears to be no generally accepted scientific basis for use of this therapy. It has never been tested in a properly controlled trial. Its use carries significant risk.*

MINERALS

**Description:** Addition of various mineral salts to diet.

**Rationale:** In almost all cases, these were empirical attempts to use agents found helpful to the general state of well-being in other diseases.

**Evaluation:** In the 1880s, associates of the French neurologist Jean Martin Charcot suggested the use of zinc phosphates in the treatment of MS. Among the early therapies for MS before 1935 were other minerals, including potassium bromide or iodide, antimony, gold, silver, mercury, arsenic, thorium, and metallic salts, which were commonly used in the treatment of many diseases. In modern times, essential minerals have been combined with vitamin supplements in a program of supplying added nutrients. There appear to be no recent reports in the scientific literature on the use of minerals alone as a specific treatment for MS. It recently was reported that there is a deficiency of manganese in people with MS. This led to the recommendation that buckwheat cakes, an excellent source of manganese, be regularly included in the diet of MS patients. No results have been reported. Zinc also has been proposed for MS, but there have been no reports of controlled studies. Another recent suggestion is long-term ingestion of potassium in the form of potassium gluconate.

**Risks/Costs:** Many minerals are toxic when ingested at any level above the traces found in normal foods.

**Conclusion:** There appears to be no clear evidence that any of these regimens should be considered effective in MS.

> *In the opinion of the Committee, there appears to be no generally accepted scientific basis for use of this therapy. It has never been tested in a properly controlled trial. Risks are undetermined.*

### CEREBROSIDES

**Description:** Dietary supplementation with fatty acids of cerebrosides from beef spinal cord.

**Rationale:** Long-chain fatty acids rapidly increase in the brain during myelination in infancy. It was suggested that dietary deficiency in such fatty acids might play a role in MS.

**Evaluation:** Fatty acids prepared from cerebrosides derived from beef spinal cord were fed to people with MS for 18 months. One sizable scientific study with matched experimental and placebo-control groups demonstrated that the experimental group did not fare any better than the control group.

**Risks/Costs:** Negligible.

**Conclusion:** On the basis of published evidence, this treatment is considered ineffective in MS.

> *In the opinion of the Committee, there appears to be no generally accepted scientific basis for use of this therapy. It has never been tested in a properly controlled trial. It is relatively free of serious adverse side effects during long-term use.*

### ALOE VERA

**Description:** Juice of the aloe vera plant; available over-the-counter; taken by mouth on a regular basis.

**Rationale:** Aloe vera juice contains vitamins, amino acids, and minerals and undoubtedly can serve as a valuable food supplement. The promotional literature for the product also asserts that it will cure a wide variety of unrelated conditions and claims that the juice has antibacterial and antiinflammatory effects.

**Evaluation:** Aloe vera juice has been taken by a number of people with MS. Anecdotal reports are available of patients who recovered from an acute attack of MS after repeatedly taking the juice. This would appear to reflect the natural history of the disease, not a real therapeutic effect. There have been no controlled trials of aloe vera juice. The FDA states, "there is no scientific evidence to support allegations that aloe vera is effective as a treatment for cancer, diabetes, or any other serious disease." Aloe vera has also been combined with other substances in a program marketed as "Herbalife." Individual patients have been reported to show favorable responses.

**Risks/Costs:** The juice generally is not harmful, but it can produce mild diarrhea and skin hypersensitivity.

**Conclusion:** Aloe vera is not recommended for use in MS.

*In the opinion of the Committee, there appears to be no generally accepted scientific basis for use of this therapy. It has never been tested in a properly controlled trial. Risks are undetermined.*

## ENZYMES

**Description:** A diet similar to the Evers diet (natural or unprocessed foods, also low in fat), supplemented with plant enzymes (Wobenzym), normal digestive enzymes, vitamins and minerals (Vitafestal), lipolytic enzymes (Bilicomb), and others (Panpur, Panzynorm).

**Rationale:** Dr. F. Schmid, a Swiss physician, has recommended a wide spectrum of enzyme substitution at mealtimes, "as long as the causal enzyme defects are not known for individual degeneration diseases." He suggests that enzyme preparations "supplement the natural supply of the foodstuffs and act as replacements in cases where a consistent diet with undenatured foodstuffs cannot be implemented."

**Evaluation:** There is no convincing evidence that people with MS have any defect in digestive function. The rationale provided does not, in fact, claim that such evidence exists. Nevertheless, the enzyme supplement is recommended by its proponents for MS and other completely unrelated diseases of the nervous system that are not known to share a common dietary mechanism. No controlled studies of such supplementation have ever been done.

**Risks/Costs:** Purchase of the recommended supplements adds significantly to the cost of a normal diet.

**Conclusion:** Enzyme supplementation is not recommended.

*In the opinion of the Committee, there appears to be no generally accepted scientific basis for use of this therapy. It has never been tested in a properly controlled trial. It is relatively free of serious adverse side effects during long-term use.*

## Useful References

- Angell M, Kassirer JP. Alternative medicine—the risks of untested and unregulated remedies. *N Engl J Med* 1998; 339:839–841.
- Bowling AC. *Alternative Medicine and Multiple Sclerosis.* New York: Demos Medical Publishing, 2001.
- Cassileth BR. *The Alternative Medicine Handbook: The Complete Reference Guide to Alternative and Complementary Therapies.* New York: W.W. Norton, 1998.
- Eisenberg DM. Advising patients who seek alternative medical therapies. *Ann Intern Med.* 1997; 127:61–69.
- Humber JM, Almeder RF (eds.). *Alternative Medicine and Ethics.* Totowa, NJ: Humana Press, 1998. Biomedical Ethics Reviews.
- Micozzi MS (ed.). Foreword by C. Everett Koop, MD. *Fundamentals of Complementary and Alternative Medicine.* New York: Churchill Livingstone, 1996.
- Wearn AM, Greenfield SM. Access to complementary medicine in general practice: Survey in one UK health authority. *J Royal Soc Med* 1998; 91:465–470.

# Index

Note: Italic (*t*) indicates a table.

Demos Medical Publishing publishes numerous books
on multiple sclerosis. These include:

*Alternative Medicine and Multiple Sclerosis*
Allen C. Bowling

*Meeting the Challenge of Progressive Multiple Sclerosis*
Patricia K. Coyle and June Halper

*Multiple Sclerosis: A Guide for the Newly Diagnosed*
Nancy J. Holland, T. Jock Murray, and Stephen C. Reingold

*Multiple Sclerosis: The Questions*
*You Have—The Answers You Need, 2nd edition*
Rosalind C. Kalb

*Multiple Sclerosis: A Guide for Families*
Rosalind C. Kalb

*Multiple Sclerosis: Your Legal Rights, 2nd edition*
Lanny E. Perkins and Sara D. Perkins

*300 Tips for Making Life with Multiple Sclerosis Easier*
Shelley Peterman Schwarz

*Employment Issues in Multiple Sclerosis*
Phillip D. Rumrill, Jr.

*Symptom Management in Multiple Sclerosis, 3rd edition*
Randall T. Schapiro

To receive additional information on these or
any of our other titles, call our toll-free number:
(800) 532-8663

Demos Medical Publishing, Inc.
386 Park Avenue South
New York, NY 10016
Phone (212) 683-0072
Fax (212) 683-0118
E-mail: orderdept@demospub.com
Web site: demosmedpub.com